Bodies Unbound

Critical Issues in Health and Medicine

Edited by Rima D. Apple, University of Wisconsin–Madison and Janet Golden, Rutgers University–Camden

Growing criticism of the U.S. healthcare system is coming from consumers, politicians, the media, activists, and healthcare professionals. Critical Issues in Health and Medicine is a collection of books that explores these contemporary dilemmas from a variety of perspectives, among them political, legal, historical, sociological, and comparative, and with attention to crucial dimensions such as race, gender, ethnicity, sexuality, and culture.

For a list of titles in the series, see the last pages of the book.

Bodies Unbound

Gender-Specific Cancer and Biolegitimacy

Piper Sledge

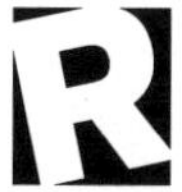

Rutgers University Press
New Brunswick, Camden, and Newark, New Jersey, and London

Library of Congress Cataloging-in-Publication Data

Names: Sledge, Piper, author.
Title: Bodies unbound: gender-specific cancer and biolegitimacy / Piper Sledge.
Description: New Brunswick, New Jersey: Rutgers University Press, 2020. | Series: Critical issues in health and medicine | Includes bibliographical references and index.
Identifiers: LCCN 2020022236 | ISBN 9781978815780 (paperback) | ISBN 9781978815797 (cloth) | ISBN 9781978815803 (epub) | ISBN 9781978815827 (pdf)
Subjects: MESH: Breast Neoplasms—psychology | Breast Neoplasms, Male—psychology | Transgender Persons | Gender Identity | Social Perception
Classification: LCC RC280.B8 | NLM WP 870 | DDC 616.99/449—dc23
LC record available at https://lccn.loc.gov/2020022236

A British Cataloging-in-Publication record for this book is available from the British Library.

∞ The paper used in this publication meets the requirements of the American National Standard for Information Sciences—Permanence of Paper for Printed Library Materials, ANSI Z39.48-1992.

www.rutgersuniversitypress.org

Manufactured in the United States of America

For Noah and Zoe

Contents

Bodies Unbound

Introduction

Cancer in the Public Imagination

The medical profession has a gender problem. This gender problem is especially prominent given that we live in an era of unprecedented access to health-related information about diseases, diagnoses, prevention, and our own genetic makeup. In May 2013, actor and humanitarian activist Angelina Jolie published an op-ed piece in the *New York Times* in which she explained her decision to get tested for BRCA (BReast CAncer gene), a genetic anomaly that significantly increases a person's lifetime risk of breast, ovarian, prostate, and pancreatic cancers. After testing positive for this condition, Jolie chose to undergo a prophylactic bilateral mastectomy, a surgery to remove both breasts, to minimize her risk of eventually developing breast cancer. She wrote, "I do not feel any less of a woman. I feel empowered that I made a strong choice that in no way diminishes my femininity" (Jolie 2013).

Jolie's essay launched a flurry of controversy, with medical professionals and other breast cancer survivors critiquing her decision. Concerns in the press and the medical community centered on three main issues: whether such surgery (often deemed "radical" in the press) was medically warranted; the "perils of over awareness" or basing medical decisions on fears about the potential development of breast cancer; and the risk of "psychological harm after having radical surgery" (Davies 2013; Ferro 2013). Jolie's account of her diagnosis and treatment, along with public criticism of her decisions by physicians, illustrates a conflict between medical authority and patient agency in medical decision-making. The heart of this conflict, as Jolie so clearly addressed, has to do with the idea that by removing breasts people may lose their femininity or their status as women. Although prophylactic mastectomy has become a standard recommendation for women diagnosed with BRCA, the impact and importance of femininity to this surgery remains contested. At the heart of this conflict is not simply the matter of medical authority, but the relationship between gender identity, embodiment, and the perpetuation of cultural ideologies of gender through the medical regulation of patient bodies. Essentially, this controversy raises the question of who gets to make choices about their bodies, under what circumstances, and for what consequences to the gender order?

Ideologies of gender are not only at play in the decisions that patients may make regarding what type of care they receive, but even whether they receive care at all for breast and gynecological cancers. In early August 2011 an array of news media outlets ran the story of twenty-six-year-old Raymond Johnson. A month earlier, Johnson, an insured tile layer, had gone to a South Carolina emergency room (ER) after finding a lump in his chest. His trip to the ER led to a diagnosis of breast cancer. Anticipating lofty medical bills, Mr. Johnson applied for a supplementary program within Medicaid created by the Breast and Cervical Cancer Prevention and Treatment Act of 2000, which provides coverage for low-income cancer patients.[1] His application was denied on the grounds that the act specifically applied only to women.

The story of Robert Eads, a transgender man denied care for ovarian and cervical cancer, was even more drastic. When Eads transitioned from female to male in the 1980s, he was no stranger to preventive gynecological care; he had given birth to two children in the 1970s. After his transition, however, he never again sought out such care, and the potential risks of "female cancers" for trans men were understudied and deemed unlikely by doctors of the time. In the mid-1990s, Eads presented at an ER at the urging of two friends because of severe vaginal bleeding, a symptom of what ultimately was diagnosed as ovarian cancer. Two dozen doctors in the region of the South where he lived refused him treatment because he was a man and therefore had the "wrong body" for preventive gynecological care (Davis 2001).

These stories are striking because of the ways that health and gender come into tension. Specifically, the study of health "permits the revelation of those elements of western cultures which bear most directly on the construction of gender and its consequences for women, men, and the larger social order" (Lewin and Olesen 1985, 19, quoted in Annandale 2009, 146). This relationship is embedded in the history of the term *gender* itself. The birth of the term "gender" occurred in the context of treatment of intersex, transgender, and other ambiguously bodied people in the 1950s (see Meyerowitz 2002; Repo 2013, 2016). However, the centrality of gender to health and medical care is not unique to trans*[2] and intersex individuals. Rather, medical care turns on assumptions about gendered bodies that become evident in provider–patient interactions that question these taken-for-granted norms. Although it has been well established that medical practice (and particularly) surgery impose a normative, binary gender order on the multiplicity of sexes possible in human beings (Davis 2015; Davis, Dewey, and Murphy 2016; Fausto-Sterling 1993, 2000; Lucal 2008; Preves 2000, 2002), I use moments of disruption in the cycle of cancer care to dig deeper into the role of medicine in perpetuating cultural ideologies of gender through the regulation of patient bodies, the ways that patients can imagine new possibilities of gendered embodiment, and the role of the medical system in legitimizing (or not) those possibilities.

In *Bodies Unbound,* I investigate the regulation of gendered bodies within the cycle of care for female cancers. I focus on the experiences of fifty-seven individuals whose bodies and gender identities do not match the medical and cultural expectations for gynecological and breast cancer prevention and care. I link together the experiences of transgender men, cisgender men, and cisgender women who all create "gender trouble" for medical professionals when their bodies or their choices concerning those bodies challenge the standards of care for these cancers and/or normative expectations for gendered bodies. The cases presented here of individuals who trouble medical protocols and expectations for gendered embodiment highlight the perpetuation of legitimate forms of gendered embodiment as well as factors that may allow us to imagine new possibilities. My central concern in this book is to understand how certain configurations of bodies and gender identities come to be understood as legitimate and intelligible through interactions with medical professionals, family, friends, and strangers.

The narrative accounts considered in this project concerning patients with the "wrong body" for gynecological and breast cancers indicate that processes of gender accountability and determination hinge on the alignment of individual identity, physical body, and normative expectations about appropriately gendered bodies. Throughout the book, I draw on empirical data to incorporate ethnomethodological theories of gender with theories of embodiment and medical regulatory power. By focusing on patients who disrupt this alignment in the context of female cancers, I raise the issue of the regulation of gendered embodiment as a critical puzzle that illustrates the ways in which taken-for-granted cultural ideologies of gender both shape and are shaped by medical interactions.

It is my intention to question the current framing of medicine as an institution of control with respect to gender and to shift the analytical focus to processes of meaning-making and value creation initiated by patients. This book is not a story about controlling doctors and individual freedom. Rather, this is a story about gender: the meanings we associate with it, and the ways in which we acquiesce, resist, imagine possibilities, and otherwise participate in these processes as patients and practitioners.

Gender, Health, and Biopower

I began this chapter with the premise that medicine—as an institution with authority over human bodies and identities, as a profession, and as space of research on the human condition—has a gender problem. If health is a means by which individuals do gender (Moore 2010) and if accomplishing an intelligible gender is necessary for achieving a livable life (Butler 2004), then this is a problem that begs for resolution. This problem is succinctly summarized across an array of research papers indicating that there are major health inequalities that track on gendered lines. This scholarship asserts that the way to solve this problem is to refute binary, categorical, and normative definitions of gender and find ways to incorporate relational, process-based understandings of gender (see Annandale [2005] 2014; Connell 2012; Hammarström et al. 2014; Springer, Hankivsky, and Bates 2012). In more basic terms, these critiques of the profession call on physicians and clinical researchers to reorient their thinking toward seeing medicine as influenced by, influencing, and deeply embedded within the gender order. Additionally, practitioners and researchers lack a clear and well-understood definition of what they actually mean when they invoke gender, because this term may deployed when researchers mean sex assigned at birth, self-identification, and the degree to which people are perceived/perceive themselves as feminine or masculine (Hart, Saperstein, Magliozzi, and Westbrook 2019).

Rather than studying the outcomes of medical care as it tracks on patient behavior, it is necessary to consider the embeddedness of gender within medicine in order to identify the moments when gender is deployed as (and thus re-created) as biopower and the factors that may contribute to resistance. In her genealogy of gender, Jemima Repo argues that "gender emerged specifically as a new *apparatus* for the regulation of the species" (2013, 240, emphasis in the original). That is, gender is *biopower*, specifically "a power over human conduct" (Fassin 2009, 45) that was created by and continues to be reinforced within medical care for the purpose of regulating bodies out of (gender) order (see also Meyerowitz 2002).

Conceptualizing gender as biopower creates a bridge between the ubiquitous concept "doing gender" (West and Zimmerman 1987) and the growing scholarship on biopolitics. I contend that it is within these interactions that resistance primarily occurs, but that the location of these interactions within medical care is particularly important given the ongoing role of the medical profession in maintaining gender as a taken-for-granted system. With this view, I am aligned with scholars who suggest that health behaviors and healthfulness are intertwined with the gender order and how individuals "do gender" (see Carpenter 2000; Moore 2010). Especially important to my understanding of participant story is the notion that not only are behaviors implicated in the doing of health and gender, but that through this doing we are actively (re)creating the very meanings of gender (see Moore 2010).

The concept of doing gender, the notion that through our daily interaction we create our own gender through accountability to cultural norms, lacks a point of origin for these norms to which we are accountable. Certainly, these norms are historically variable and become enmeshed in institutions and the minutia of daily life, but the centrality of interactions to creating this meaning cannot be overstated. The move to understand gender as biopower not only identifies the historical emergence of the term but also provides an explanation for why the pressure to be accountable to gender norms is so great and difficult to change. The association of gender with biopower also leads to a more effective place to begin understanding the factors that may contribute to change.

As Michel Foucault famously argued, where there is power there is resistance (1978), but where might resistance occur given the power of gender over life itself? Much of the scholarship building on the concept of biopower turns on the role of the state while obscuring microlevel interactions. Two threads in the scholarship emerging from the concept of biopower are particularly instructive for unraveling the tension that gender creates in medical care: biocitizenship and biolegitimacy.[3] *Biocitizenship* refers to the notion that corporeality is essential to personal and interactive practices of identity and that individuals as citizens have a set of biological responsibilities regarding health behaviors and education (Rose and Novas 2005). Given advances in medical and biological knowledge, individuals are now more than ever expected to behave in ways that ensure the overall enhancement of health and the prolongment of the life span. Despite the potential possibilities that attention to biopolitics and biocitizenship create, the biological presuppositions that underpin biocitizenship have "shaped conception of what it means to be a citizen, and underpinned distinctions between actual, potential, troublesome, and impossible citizens" (Rose 2007, 132).

Because people are expected to seek out and make decisions based on knowledge about health and related practices, biocitizens are empowered in the ways promoted by the women's health movement of the 1960s and 1970s. That is, they are expected to have the knowledge to make their own decisions and have those decisions be respected by medical professionals, but this ability is constrained by government structures that need to regulate social order and also by the fact that biocitizenship turns on an implicit distinction between men and women that is taken to be biological fact. In the context of biocitizenship, a person's accountability to gender ideology cannot be separated from biomedical imaginaries of embodiment. To be a good biocitizen requires adopting certain health behaviors or bodily practices, including submitting to medical exams. This care is predicated on differences between male and female bodies that are naturalized through interactions and legitimized through the institutional practices of the medical profession. Thus, biocitizenship becomes "those citizenship projects that have linked their conceptions of citizens to beliefs about the biological existence of human beings, as individuals, *as men and women,* as families and lineages, as communities, as populations and races, and as a species" (Rose 2007, 132, emphasis added).

Much engagement with biopolitics leaves out the relationship between everyday life and politics. Sociologist Didier Fassin (2009) attempts to fill this gap through the concept of *biolegitimacy.* Bringing this relationship to the fore allows for attention to what lives people may live and the creation of meaning and value in those daily experiences. With this focus, biopower becomes a normalizing factor in the daily lives of people and biolegitimacy as "the power of life" becomes a way to conceptualize "the sort of life people may or may not live" (Fassin 2009, 49). Biolegitimacy then refers to the power of everyday life in creating meaning and value, but it must be held in relation to the forces of biopower if that power is to be resisted or if new meanings can inform the workings of biopower.

Through their health behaviors and the interactions that inform and emerge from them, biocitizens buy into or reject normative ideas of healthfulness, but they also have the responsibility to become knowledgeable about their bodies and are empowered to act upon that knowledge in daily life, including interactions with medical professionals. Behaving in ways that fail to align with certain expectations renders one troublesome as a citizen and as a patient. This determination of a person as a troublesome citizen is bound up with the biopower of gender to control and regulate individuals. If gender can be biopower (e.g., power over life), can it also be biolegitimacy (e.g., the power of life and a process of meaning creation in everyday life)? I attest that *gendered biolegitimacy* brings greater focus to the ways in which embodiment, power, and legitimacy are (re)produced in everyday life within the context of normative structures. Chiefly, I argue that the specific addition of gender to the concept of biolegitimacy suggests that this normative force is not only about how people live, but also about what sorts of bodies they may have and how those bodies become legitimate in our own minds and those of others around us. Further, using the language of biolegitimacy allows for consideration of how the meaning and value of gender may be reproduced or reimagined within daily life while also impacting the locus of gender's biopower: the medical community.

If gender is biopower, then it is upheld not only by medical professionals but also by the imperatives of biocitizenship. Biocitizenship also creates a tension between the institution upholding the system and the subjects who exist within it. The agency and subjectivity afforded to biocitizens empowers patients to imagine new embodiments that may disrupt normative meanings of gender and to request that medical professionals support them in making these possibilities reality. These new possibilities are not automatically afforded biolegitimacy—that is, recognition as viable, visible, and acceptable by the medical community. Biolegitimacy is just not a state matter but a medical matter as well, because medical authorities have access to technologies that these troublesome patients require to construct bodies that make sense to them given the disruptions of illness. Gendered biolegitimacy is about how medical authorities attempt to wrangle troublesome biocitizens back into the order of gender and how biocitizens stretch the limits of gender itself.

I intend my use of gendered biolegitimacy to expand beyond Aihwa Ong's original use of the term in 2011. Ong used "gendered bio-legitimacy" in reference to the right of female migrants to a "healthy and unthreatened body" (2011, 42). Like much of the scholarship on biopolitics, gendered bio-legitimacy here does not turn to everyday experience but rather equates health with "the good life" and the importance of women as "life-givers and life-nurturers" (Ong 2011, 42). The term describes the right to health that should be afforded to people deemed female based on the physical capacity of bearing and birthing children and the associated expectation that these same people will bear the burden of supporting the life and health of others beyond the womb. This approach takes gender and health as always already defined. I approach gender as a puzzle and consider health to be a changing and conflicted term that also functions as biopower (see Metzl and Kirkland 2010).

My use of the term gendered biolegitimacy unites the concepts of biolegitimacy with the notion that gender is biopower, and it links them to the responsibilities conferred to individuals via biocitizenship to consider the ways that biopower confers meaning and value through ideologies of gender. That is, this is a kind of spiraling process where biocitizens can confront medical professionals (as gatekeepers and upholders of gender as biopower) to advocate for the legitimacy of different configurations of bodies and gender identities, thus effecting changes in gender itself. Fundamentally, the concept of gendered biolegitimacy allows for the theorizing of resistance to normative expectations of gendered bodies and the governing power of medical authorities. If we seek to address gender inequality or to open the possibilities of what livable lives may be, then we need to consider the ways that regularly occurring medical interactions between providers and patients can intervene in the perpetuation of gender as biopower.

The Case of Gynecological and Breast Cancers

Gynecological and breast cancers present an ideal context in which to identify the impact of normative ideologies of gender and to imagine new possibilities for embodiment because they allow for the examination of patient experiences and the embeddedness of gender at every point in the medical cycle of care—the care of these cancers turns on managing the threat to and restoring femininity (see Ericksen 2008; Potts 2000; Sulik 2011). Further, at each point in the cycle of care (i.e., early detection/prevention, diagnosis, treatment, and recovery), biomedical intervention is standard, and the details of diagnosis and treatment of the diseases in question are highly specialized (although well known to many patients). Because of their deeply specialized knowledge, this dynamic places physicians in a position of relative power over the bodies and lives of patients. Still, patients have unprecedented access to knowledge about diagnosis and treatment options. This knowledge and the ever-increasing influence of social media and social networks provide opportunities for resisting the power of physicians as sole decision-makers.

"Female" cancers are particularly well situated as a context for exploring how bodies and gender relate and become visible and legitimate in daily life through medical interventions. Bodies assigned female at birth are routinely subjected to medical screenings to catch cancer as early as possible. The Papanicolaou (Pap) test, which involves the extraction of cervical cells via scraping, is the only medical intervention that can identify precancerous cells; early detection thus effectively prevents cervical cancers. Mammograms, administered for early detection of breast cancer, are a part of standard medical care for women although there is some debate over the ideal timing for mammograms. The test for BRCA was the first genetic test to assess cancer risk, although BRCA tests remain a recommendation for some patients rather than a standard for all to follow. "Female" cancers are unique in that the medical community generally agrees that these tests are important components of cancer care for people assigned female at birth, while medical exams for "male" cancers are much less effective.[4]

These cancers become enmeshed with hegemonic gender norms because they grow in body parts with a great deal of symbolic importance for the meaning of gender (see Spade 2003). Breasts are especially "celebrated as the principal symbol of womanhood, motherhood, and female sexuality" (Sulik 2011, 14–15). Relying on normative conceptions of femininity based in a binary gender system serves to "recast the uncertainty of illness into something more manageable and valued" (Sulik 2011, 74). In everyday life, breast cancer awareness slogans such as "Save the Ta Tas" and "Save Second Base," and the proliferation of pink paraphernalia in October indicate threats to female embodiment and heterosexuality and communicate that reinforcing femininity is the means by which to recover from this disease. With the "Turn It Teal" and "Teal Heels" campaigns (represented by a teal high-heel shoe with gynecological cancer facts) and slogans that implore women to "check their box" and "help the hoo-hahs," gynecological cancer activism draws on similar narrative tools. Activism for these cancers, primarily diagnosed in cisgender women, draws on tropes of femininity to mobilize research funding and public awareness.

Breast and gynecological cancers are unique windows into the everyday medical interactions that we routinely experience and the role these interactions play in maintaining or resisting structures of gender and sexuality. Gender-specific cancers show how hegemonic gender norms shape public discourse as well as how women and men respond to their diagnosis and treatment options (see, for example, Casper and Carpenter 2008; Hesse-Biber 2014; Klawiter 2008; Oliffe 2009; Sulik 2011). Given the constraints of the gender system, patients often behave in predictable ways; we expect to see people maintain the system. But what might resistance look like and what are potential threats to the system? What other possibilities exist for gendered embodiment? Interpersonal interactions that trouble the system are the foundations for understanding change. If we seek to alter the reality of gender inequality in medical care, we must begin research at these points of gender trouble because they illustrate the often invisible influence of cultural ideologies of gender on medical care. Analyzing the way these ideologies are made real through medical interactions allows us to better understand how these ideologies in turn shape gender inequalities in health.

Female cancers allow for the examination of gender ideologies in all phases of the medical cycle of care because medical interventions are standard at every point in the cycle. This cycle is not specific to cancer. Rather, it is the cycle of prevention and treatment that characterizes medical care. In both the cultural imagination and in medical care, the narrative of female cancer assumes a "right body" for care that aligns with a female identified, cisgender woman with normative desires for her body's appearance. When a patient does not meet these assumptions, they create gender trouble for health care providers. Interview data from such troubling patients identifies the importance of normative expectations for gendered bodies to medical care and the ways in which such care reinforces the legitimacy of these expectations.

Project Design and Overview

Within the collective cultural imagination generally and in medical care specifically, the narrative around breast and gynecological cancers turns on stereotypes of femininity and female sexuality: the "right patient" for care is a cisgender, female-identified, heterosexual woman with normative desires for her body's appearance. To understand the ways in which gender shapes medical decision-making, I interviewed individuals whose bodies, desires for their bodies, and/or gender identities do not match the medical and culturally normative expectations for gynecological and breast cancer care: transgender men, cisgender men, cisgender women who choose prophylactic mastectomy, and cisgender women who live flat after mastectomy.[5] These are people whose bodies are out of order with respect to gender and thus make clear the ways that the medical profession attempts to put them back in order—that is, in alignment with normative expectations of gender—thus reinforcing the biopower of these ideologies.

I purposely chose to focus on patient experiences rather than on providers because these stories are those that are left out of the public discourse on these cancers. Instead of searching for "true experience," the interviews I conducted provide insight into the processes by which individuals understand themselves and their social worlds; as a result, they also reveal how those social worlds come into being (Connell 2005). Although this process occurs in interactions between patients and providers, I chose to begin with the patients because theirs are the bodies implicated in these interactions and they are the ones who must live with the decisions.

I conducted in-depth, narrative interviews to explore the details of participants' experiences and the ways in which they made sense of these experiences. The interviews ranged from 45 minutes to 2.5 hours and were conducted in person, by video conferencing (via Skype or FaceTime), and over the phone, depending on participant's location and preference. The participants ranged in age from 22 to 71 years. I recruited participants through social media groups for transgender men, men with breast cancer, women who are BRCA positive ("previvors"), and women who refuse breast reconstruction ("live flat"). I also identified participants through a snowball sample, beginning with both people in my own social networks and from participants recruited through social media. (Appendix A contains further details about participant demographics.)

The participants here represent a series of cases that highlight the problem of gender in medical care and the ways in which gender functions as biopower. With the exception of BRCA-positive previvors, medical protocols do not exist to accommodate the bodies, identities, or desires of participants in this study. As the example of Angelina Jolie shows, it is only recently that the medical community has incorporated standards to support BRCA-positive women in choosing mastectomy. Still, living flat after a diagnosis of BRCA or breast cancer remains outside the normative scope of medical care. Taken together, these cases set up a series of contrasts in the ability of patients to determine the relationship between their gender and their bodies in the service of achieving health. These comparisons form the basis of the chapters to follow and illustrate the ongoing role of the medical profession in maintaining the social order through the regulation of gendered bodies. It is important to note early on that participants in my research represent a conservative test of the problems of gender and the body for medical practice and gender theory. This is a privileged sample: white, middle-class, employed, insured, and well-educated.[6] These are the individuals who should have the most power to advocate their desires in medical interactions, but my research shows that this is not the case.

This book explores how patients experience gender in these moments of uncertainty and how they perceive the response of the medical community. It does not actually matter whether these perceptions are "true," in the sense the providers would corroborate the narratives of the participants. The truth of these accounts lies with the teller: lay people have too long been silenced, dismissed, and ignored by those with certain kinds of expertise and the power that extends from that knowledge.

What matters is not actually what the doctors say to patients or how doctors interpret the advice they give. We are conditioned to only believe experts; but experience also provides expertise, and the experiences of one's own body are very real. A patient's perception of an interaction has everything to do with how treatment will progress. Rather than the medical community trying to find ways to convince patients to do what they say and that "doctor knows best" (i.e., patient compliance concerns), the medical community needs to learn to listen to their patients and adapt to what they hear—not to convince, cajole, or guilt patients into doing what providers think is best based on standards of care built on assumptions about gender and acceptable embodiment. Instead, providers need to actually hear what patients are saying and work with patients to live their lives as they wish to live them, not as providers think they should be lived. By focusing on patients who disrupt this alignment in the context of female cancers, I raise the issue of the regulation of gendered embodiment as a critical puzzle that illustrates the ways in which taken-for-granted cultural ideologies of gender both shape and are shaped by medical interactions.

Chapter Overview

This book tells a story about how bodies, gender, and the perceptions of others go together in both expected and unexpected ways. It is also a story of how this relationship becomes intelligible through the experiences of individuals, as well as of how medical professionals use their authority over bodies to legitimize certain combinations of bodies and genders. It is a story of conformity, rebellion, and possibility. It is an illustration of how we become who we are in a neoliberal culture marked by a paradoxical desire to be at once an individual yet to also be a recognizable and accepted member of society. It is a story about creating possibilities for livable lives that account for experiences that are outside the cultural norms that govern gender. The setting for this story is an increasingly medicalized world, in which individuals are interpellated to be biocitizens—that is, to control their bodies, health, and medical fate—but only insofar as those behaviors coincide with accepted medical knowledge and culturally prescribed behaviors.

The next four chapters of the book are organized by key points in the cycle of cancer care: prevention/diagnosis, treatment, and recovery. The first three chapters emphasize the factors influencing their experiences while the fourth chapter engages with elective surgeries as powerful forces in maintaining and questioning the workings of biopower in cancer care. Within each of these phases of care, different groups of participants explain their experiences of being out of place and troubling the taken-for-granted assumptions upon which care in each phase is predicated. In each chapter, I juxtapose experiences from different groups of patients in order to magnify the influence of normative ideologies of gender on the decision- and meaning-making processes that participants undertake. When I shift to a direct focus on elective surgical decision-making for these cancers, I draw on the arguments of the previous chapters to point directly to medical processes that prioritize gender over empirically based medicine and patient-centered care.

In chapter 1, "Entering Enemy Territory?," I compare the narratives of transgender and cisgender men as they navigate women-centered spaces of cancer care in order to prevent and diagnose gynecological and breast cancer. Drawing on the experiences of transgender men seeking gynecological care and cisgender men seeking breast cancer care, I develop the argument that assumptions about gendered bodies are at the heart of medical practice yet are problematic for patients. The way these men make sense of the health care they receive reflects the ambiguous relationship of body parts to gender identity and the ways in which normative masculinity is deployed differentially by providers, depending on whether a patient is transgender or cisgender, to manage male bodies in the distinctly feminized spaces of breast cancer care.

Participant stories of prophylactic mastectomy are the focus of chapter 2, "Choosing Mastectomy." Here, patient perceptions of health risks, interpersonal relationships, and personal identity are revealed in the ways in which cisgender women make sense of their decisions to undergo prophylactic mastectomy as a preventative option after being diagnosed with BRCA or breast cancer. Women with BRCA and women with breast cancer described different responses from health care providers when seeking prophylactic mastectomies. Although women in these groups have similar concerns for their health and the treatment they think they need, some women experienced tension with their medical providers. In this chapter, women explain the ways that gender ideologies seep into their decisions about treatments as well as the recommendations they received from their providers.

In chapter 3, "Returning to Normal," the experiences of both women and cisgender men in recovering from breast cancer intersect with ideas about normalcy and bodily integrity. Here, I discuss the various external forces that influence women's reconstruction decisions. I examine how participants make sense of their bodies after cancer and how they come to understand their bodies as authentic, normal, and beautiful, regardless of their treatment experiences. Although reconstruction options are rarely presented to cisgender men, both they and cisgender women struggle with similar factors as they heal from breast cancer treatments.

Decision-making for elective surgeries related to breast and gynecological cancer is the focus of chapter 4, "Ideologies of Gender in Surgical Cancer Care." These surgeries illustrate the ways in which patients and providers rely on frames of gender to determine whether a given surgery is an appropriate option for cancer prevention or care. These cases explain how medical interactions are shaped by and thus reproduce ideologies of gender through the bodies of patients. The medical interactions leading to these surgeries can be particularly fraught and may bring to the fore the ways in which medical care is implicated in reproducing gendered biolegitimacy. A condensed version of this chapter was first published in *Social Science & Medicine* (Sledge 2019).

Together, these cases comprise a unique perspective into processes by which identity, bodies, and medical care are relationally constituted, and they demonstrate why certain bodies create such "trouble" for the institution of medicine. The ways in which trans men, cis men, and cis women navigate medical care for body parts imbued with gendered meanings underscores that medical care in practice, policy, and theory needs new tools for making sense of gender in order to improve patient access to and experiences of medical care. Throughout, I argue that medical care is largely shaped by commonly held beliefs about what it means to be a woman or a man and how those meanings map onto and shape the physical body. These beliefs, on the part of providers, shape gender. Gender is not a variable determining access to care and health outcomes, nor is it an individual attribute. Rather, medical practices are embedded within the gender system; as such, they are influenced by cultural ideologies of gender. Medical care is shaped by ideas about gender while also reproducing those beliefs through the bodies of patients.

Medical care is instrumental in determining which combinations of bodies and identities are legitimate or socially intelligible. By using medical language to justify normative expectations of gendered bodies, not only do medical interactions regulate patient bodies, but they also mark certain bodies as legitimate and others as illegitimate or wrong. The narrative accounts considered here of patients with the wrong body for gynecological and breast cancers indicate that processes of gender accountability and determination hinge on the alignment of individual identity, physical body, and normative expectations about appropriately gendered bodies. By focusing on patients who disrupt this alignment, I raise the issue of the regulation of gendered embodiment as a catalyst for critical inquiry and a response to critiques of medicine put forth by gender theorists. I argue that we must better understand gender as an embodied process in order to rethink the ways in which the gender system is re-created, resisted, and reimagined as well as to more clearly theorize the linkages between levels of analysis in the gender system.

Chapter 1

Entering Enemy Territory?

The stories in this chapter recount varying relationships between men's bodies, identities, masculinity, and femininity. Although normative expectations of gendered embodiment link breasts, uteri, and ovaries with women and femininity, and penises and testicles with men and masculinity, the reality is that these relationships are much more ambiguous than many would like to believe.

When designing this research, I naively assumed that men would explain experiences of breast and gynecological care as threatening to their identities. Instead, their stories reveal that men experience this care differently based on gradations in their position of "wrong" embodiment. That is, cisgender men described a lack of alignment between their bodies and medical protocols, and transgender men described a lack of alignment between their identities and normative expectations about men's' bodies. For both groups of men, this lack of alignment created a degree of trouble in the health care interaction that required resolution through the management of men's bodies, identities, and the perceptions of others in the clinic. By understanding this dynamic, the stories shared by these men expose processes of gendered biolegitimacy.

In this chapter, I focus on the experiences of transgender and cisgender men seeking diagnoses and early detection care for breast and gynecological cancers. The chapter begins with the experience of seeking care and follows men as they enter clinical spaces designated for women, describe their perceptions of obtaining care, and their thoughts about being men in women's spaces.

Suspicions, Seeking Care, and Diagnosis

When I asked Frank about being diagnosed with breast cancer, he said, "I'm a man who was just told you have [breast] cancer. And I am floored. . . . It was just like someone hit me with a two-by-four . . . I'm sitting there going, 'Holy shit. I'm a man [laughs], and I have breast cancer.'" This was a common sentiment among cis men after receiving a breast cancer diagnosis. Even those who suspected that they had cancer expressed degrees of surprise at their diagnosis. Trans men, like some of the cis men, had somewhat vague concerns about cervical, ovarian, and uterine cancer risk, but many reported a degree of unconcern and let the relative invisibility of these parts justify not seeking preventive health care. As Zach explained, "I usually just ignore that part of my body."

For most men, breast cancer is unthinkable, and gynecological cancers are not concerning, unless a person experiences alarming symptoms. This is not entirely surprising. Male breast cancer makes up only 1 percent of diagnoses, even though the incidence has been increasing in the United States since 1978 (Speirs et al. 2010; Speirs and Shaaban 2009). Public awareness that men can get breast cancer has been limited, and clinical research on breast cancer in men remains sparse, thus contributing to the unthinkability of male breast cancer. There is also a relative lack of data about the risk of gynecological cancers for trans men although data does suggest that part of this risk is due to trans people being less likely than cis people to receive preventive screenings (James et al. 2016; Rollston 2019). For both breast and cervical cancers, screening technologies (i.e. mammograms and Pap tests) and standards of care exist that are highly effective at diagnosing physical symptoms early in disease onset or even before they become cancerous. However, these technologies are not standard care for men.

Research on men and health suggests that cultural ideologies of masculinity may render men less likely to seek care (see Bish et al. 2005; Courtenay 2000; Doucleff 2013; Oliffe 2009; Pinkhasov et al. 2010; Rosenfeld and Faircloth 2006; Stibbe 2004; Vaidya, Partha, and Karmakar 2012; Watson 2000). Cis men in this study largely supported this research. Ezra stated that he rarely went to the doctor because "I have no complaints. . . . If I don't have a physical complaint, I just don't go to the doctor." Similarly, Henry stated that he visited a doctor only "to treat a broken collarbone or other [sports] related injury" and emphasized his overall sense of robust health: "I was always super healthy. I didn't realize that I was particularly vulnerable to anything." Tim expressed a clear link between avoiding medical care and masculinity. "I think it's just us being men. We think that you know, oh, nothing is going to bring me down. You know, I'm healthy as an ox, and unless we feel like we're on our deathbed, we don't go to the doctor."

James was one of the few cis men who advocated regular medical care. He expressed a deep disdain for men relatives who "talk with a kind of bravado, 'Oh, I never go to the doctor.'" "Bravado" here serves as a code for masculinity. When imitating this relative, James's voice dropped an octave, and he added a sort of swagger to his voice. Still, James reiterated the sentiment that medical visits were important primarily if something was wrong. "I mean, if something ain't right, get it checked out. That's my philosophy." The habit of avoiding medical care and the lack of widespread recognition that breast cancer is more than just a women's disease can impact the care men receive.

Some of the trans men in this study were very clear about their concerns going into medical exams that are designed with an expectation of women patients. Isaac explained that after multiple experiences where health care providers struggled to look past his identity as trans and to provide appropriate medical care, he constantly worried about the consequences of failing to align with provider expectations of embodiment.

> What I'm afraid of is when people are surprised by the fact that my body is not what they expect, that it literally, like, shuts down their ability to process information in their brain [laughs]. Like, it becomes something that's totally all-consuming. I don't know if this is actually what's happening. I'm just postulating. But, like, their ability to then ask relevant medical questions, to provide me with information that's necessary, to communicate with other medical staff at a level where they were previously before finding out that I was trans, it just goes down. So I think that because it's such a surprise to people it hinders their ability to function as medical professionals. And so my fear is, I'm going to go in, they're going to get freaked out, and then they just won't be able to do their jobs in the way that I absolutely need them to do their jobs. So that's what my fear is.

For some trans men, this kind of fear shaped gynecological care into what Erik described as a "violent act" because of the forced disruption between body and identity that can result from microaggressions and outright discrimination. For Gabe, fear and past experiences where providers exhibited an inability to reconcile his identity and his embody led to a vehement rejection of gynecological care.

> All things being equal, you can have nine women come in, and there's some kind of understanding and appreciation that you're helping me to

> stay healthy. From a transgender patient [perspective], you're not. There's an anxiety and a pain level and a discomfort level walking in. There's a tension to the body, and it's resistant to the care that's being offered, I would suggest to you, and so that's gonna present in the exam. It will be more difficult to do what you do and know that we're fighting you, [laughs] at least I am. I'm fighting whatever you do, and here's the thing about that—that's why we don't go to the doctor. I'm gonna speak because I've heard these voices, all right, and most of us would rather *die* than to be treated for that kind of care, like gynecological or mammograms. We won't go for those exams. We'd rather die.

Despite the pressures of masculinity and fear of discrimination or poor treatment, the men in this study did seek preventative and diagnostic care, even if they delayed it for a time. In doing so, they directly confronted the ways in which ideologies of gender shape the spaces, medical technologies, and clinical exams for breast and gynecological care. Two factors emerged as the primary motivations for seeking medical attention: unusual physical symptoms and the urging of women friends and family.

Unusual Physical Symptoms

Both trans and cis men described physical symptoms as key catalysts for seeking medical attention. These symptoms included pain, discharge, and lumps. Before their breast cancer diagnosis, most cis men in this study noticed some kind of physical abnormality on their chests. Henry felt an unusual pain when putting on a messenger bag; Ezra felt a lump behind his nipple; Tim experienced "yellow-orange-ish discharge out of [his] nipple"; and Frank, a long-distance runner, noticed irregularities in the normal chafing he experienced on runs. Frank said, "I was a runner, and every now and again a man, when he runs, tends to bleed from his nipples, and that's what happened to me particularly on my half-marathon runs. And I noticed that my right nipple started looking funky . . . like it may have a blister on it, or it was changing shape or something."

Although most trans men described their experiences with more routine preventive care and thus did not seek care for these reasons, two trans men in the study recounted similar sorts of experiences. Peter ended up in the emergency room concerned that his "vagina was pouring out rivers of unidentified fluids," and Chris sought gynecological care after experiencing severe and inexplicable pelvic pain.

Even with these acute symptoms, some men, particularly cis men, delayed care. Ezra, for example, "watched [the lump] for a while," and Tim waited "for a year to a year and a half" before seeing a doctor about fluid from his nipple. Owen noticed a lump while in the shower, and he was concerned because his mother had died of breast cancer at age thirty-seven. Nevertheless, he chose to wait until his annual physical to ask his doctor about the lump.

> I was going to see my primary care doctor in a couple of weeks anyways so I—when I saw him, we did our appointment, and I was just getting ready to leave and I said, "Well, I got this lump in my chest." And he said, "Oh, take your shirt off, let me see," and you know, he checked, and he said, "Yeah, there is something there." He told me later that he looked down at my chart and when he saw the family history that my mother died of breast cancer at thirty-seven, a little light went on, and he said, "I want you to see a surgeon."

It was unclear from our interview whether Owen would have postponed medical care had he not already had an appointment scheduled. Although his delay of a couple of weeks may not have been medically significant, Owen described his actions as delaying care. Henry's reticence to seek care was even more surprising: he not only had a family history of breast cancer but had an uncle who had died from the disease.

> I went home, and I looked down, and there was a lump on my chest. I kind of freaked out but not seriously . . . I kind of blew it off for about two or three days . . . I mean look at me. I blew it off. I didn't even bother noticing it till I was stage 2B, and I'm a prime candidate.[1] I mean I was aware, keenly aware, of the fact that men get breast cancer because of my uncle, and yet I didn't run to the doctor in a panic. I blew it off for a few days.

Waiting a few days to seek medical attention is not necessarily unusual. What is notable in Henry's case is that the reason behind the delay was his assumption that any breast abnormality in men is probably nothing. Thus, ideologies of masculinity may influence a man's timeline for decision-making even when they have knowledge about male breast cancer due to family history. These norms set a standard for men to be independent, in control of their bodies, and to reject help (Connell 1995; Courtenay 2000; Oliffe 2006).

The Encouragement of Women

Generally, symptoms and risk factors were not enough to inspire cis men to seek care. For cis men, breast cancer was largely unthinkable; for trans men, they could imagine cancer but balanced their fear of cancer with their concerns about seeking care. For cis and trans men alike, women friends and family were important catalysts for seeking care.

Like many men, Frank described his wife as being "very concerned" about the changes in his body. Upon discovering a lump in his chest, Henry "kind of freaked out, but not seriously." His wife was the instigator of care, telling him "you gotta get it checked." Ed found his lump after a woman friend urged him, via e-mail, to do self-exams. She herself had found a lump in her breast that turned out to be malignant after another friend had encouraged her to perform self-exams. Ed's friend subsequently sent an e-mail to all her friends explaining her diagnosis and encouraging them to do self-exams. He explained, "Normally the response to that is one would expect women to be responsive to that, but I [decided to] check myself now. [I found] a very small lump, about the size of a grain of sand, or I'd described as a pine nut frequently. I told my wife, and she encouraged me to have it examined, and I did so."

Women partners were integral to the decisions of some trans men as well. Joe, for example, had studiously avoided gynecological care until his wife encouraged him to have a routine screening after learning about his family history of endometriosis and cancer. Joe was unenthusiastic but submitted to his first gynecological exam to appease his spouse and was grateful that she was "right in the room, holding [his] hand." Other trans men reported bringing a friend with them to reduce some of the tension brought about by being a man submitting to a gynecological exam. More commonly, trans men described seeking preventative gynecological care as a matter of routine and attributed this behavior to their overall interest in healthfulness (that of themselves and of sexual partners), family connections to the health care industry, or family cancer history. Isaac, for example, explained that his consistent pursuit of gynecological care was motivated by personal and family history: "I had had ovarian cysts. I come from a family of endometriosis, and my mom had also had precancerous tumors in her uterus where she had a hysterectomy when she was really young." Gynecological cancer was thus very real, and the experience of his mother was a major factor in Isaac's decision to find accepting gynecologists.

For many men in this study, health care occurred at the urging of their wives, who took on the stereotypically feminine role of medical gatekeepers (see Read and Gorman 2010). It is often through women's encouragement that men decide to eventually seek medical attention and act in accordance with gender ideologies that set women up as the link between families and medical institutions. Health practices are divided along gendered lines in ways that establish a normative standard in which women support healthfulness by facilitating medical care, while men hold a culturally encouraged and potentially false belief in their own robustness and invulnerability. The urging of women friends and family members aided in legitimating men's need for what is normally considered women's health care. By virtue of their status as women, these people in the lives of the men I interviewed helped normalize the experience.

Delays in Diagnosis

Even when men have sought care after noticing strange symptoms, at the behest of women in their lives, or because their understanding of family medical history indicated they may be at increased risk for certain cancers, they struggled to find physicians who would take them seriously. Chris, a transgender man in his early twenties, explained that he had gone for his first Papanicolaou (Pap) test two years before our interview. He told me that he made the decision to seek care essentially to screen for human papillomavirus (HPV) for his own and his sexual partner's safety. His first Pap test was abnormal, and Chris was told that there was no need to worry for three years. A year after this test, Chris sought care for abdominal pain immediately after it began, yet it took him five months to find a physician who would take him seriously.

> I was feeling pain, sort of in my lower abdomen, pelvic area, what have you. . . . Between February and June [of 2013] I saw my primary care four times. Three of the times, he told me I was having gas, and the fourth time he basically told me I was making it up. He said there was nothing wrong, there was no pain, and that I needed to stop coming in for that reason. And then, in early June, I was in the ER [emergency department] because of the pain. I had to do a follow up with my doctor, but he was out of town for three weeks, so I ended up seeing a nurse practitioner. The nurse practitioner said, "Oh! This is a real problem. I'm gonna get you in to see a specialist."

Chris ended up back in the ER twice before his appointment with the gynecologist he was referred to. During Chris' time in the ER, he submitted to magnetic resonance imaging (MRI) scans, computed tomography (CT) scans, and external ultrasounds, none of which were able to clearly show his ovaries or uterus. Chris declined an internal pelvic exam after the hospital staff consistently misgendered him. He explained, "I was . . . not treated like a dude during my hospital visit at all. [Providers] do not ask your pronouns. If you told them you prefer this name, they will not respect you. [They will say,] outright, 'No I'm not allowed to call you that. No, I don't even want to.'"

When Chris finally saw the gynecologist, she told him that after receiving abnormal test results, he should have been tested again six months later. The gynecologist eventually found a mass and advised Chris to have a hysterectomy. Chris's experience of being dismissed by physicians initially and being misgendered is not uncommon. The most well-documented reason that trans men avoid or delay preventive screenings are related to concerns about encountering discriminatory health care and microaggressions (Cochran, Peavy, and Cauce 2007; Lurie 2005; Nordmarken and Kelly 2014).

The situation is not much better for cis men concerning the degree to which their concerns about breast cancer are taken seriously by providers. Medical students are often taught the following adage as they begin clinical training: "When you hear hoofbeats, look for horses, not zebras." Aspiring physicians are taught to focus on the most likely diagnosis for a group of symptoms, rather than the more unique possibilities. For men with breast cancer, this can lead to delays in diagnosis. Henry was worried about this tendency because he had "heard [about doctors who] blow off" other men with breast cancer. Henry went on to say that, in his opinion, the aggressive nature of male breast cancer is attributable to physicians' discounting breast cancer during the differential diagnosis.[2] "There is a danger in the medical community, particularly in smaller communities or with older doctors, where they go, 'Oh, it's probably just a cyst,' and I've met people in talking about that, men who were all the way at stage 4 before they're actually diagnosed even though they had gone to medical professionals in advance. That's just tragic."

Tim's story is another example of doctors downplaying the possibility of a man with breast cancer. Tim was diagnosed at a younger age than most men who have breast cancer; he noticed his lump as a teenager while stretching. When he mentioned the lump during a varsity sports physical, the team physician dismissed his concerns: "[He told me], 'It's probably just calcium build up. You're going through puberty. Your body is changing. It should go away over the next few weeks or months.' It never did." Tim brought up the lump again a year later and was told to come back if it changed in size. After college, when he secured a full-time job with health benefits, he again sought medical attention. Tim's new doctor was suspicious because the lump had been present for more than five years. It is important to recognize that if Tim were a high school-aged woman and approached a physician with a lump, it is likely her concerns would be taken seriously and breast cancer would be considered, even though breast cancer is rarely diagnosed in women this young.[3] For a high school-aged woman, breast cancer is never a "zebra" during differential diagnosis because she always will have the "right" body (and gender) for breast cancer. Men, especially young men, statistically have the wrong body for the disease. Tim could have been diagnosed with breast cancer or a condition like fibroadenoma, which can become cancerous.[4] In either case, had he been a woman there is a good possibility that he would have been treated early and the growth of a malignant tumor would have been prevented.

Although his diagnosis did not take five years to receive, Frank also faced difficulties convincing his doctor to seriously consider breast cancer as a possibility. When he asked his primary care doctor to examine his chest, the doctor said, "It's probably nothing; I'll send you to a surgeon if you want." Subsequently, the surgeon told Frank the same thing: "It's probably nothing." The surgeon's conviction that there was nothing to be concerned about prevented him from performing diagnostic tests. A month later, Frank returned, and the surgeon finally acquiesced to a biopsy that led to a cancer diagnosis.

Even when physicians take the breast cancer concerns of men seriously, often the potential severity of the diagnosis is minimized. Owen's primary care physician believed that the lump was not a major cause for concern, despite Owen's family history of breast cancer. This physician did send Owen to a surgeon, but he minimized the likely outcome: "He said at worst they'll do a lumpectomy and take it out and send it to the lab, and you'll be done with it, and I said, 'Oh, okay.'" The response of physicians is somewhat like the masculine bravado James recounted earlier. Sometimes, both men and their physicians believe that physical abnormalities in the chest are unworthy of attention. Both may believe that men are largely invulnerable to breast cancer and that there must be a better explanation than cancer.

The downplaying of breast cancer and gynecological issues by some men and some of their physicians is, in my assessment, a result of the statistical and narrative framing of breasts, ovaries, cervixes, and uteri as female body parts, subject to women's diseases. In their initial discounting of the possibility of illness, physicians and patients reaffirm the power of ideas about masculinity in shaping men's approach to health care and the actual care they receive, resulting in potentially dire consequences for their diagnosis and treatment. These reifications of cultural norms pathologize masculinity as risky for men's health and mark men's bodies as wrong for breast and gynecological care because cancer prevention and diagnosis in these body parts is linked to women and femininity culturally and medically. Thus, the care-seeking behaviors and the reactions of providers described by men are not simply about masculinity. Rather, the act of seeking care may also constitute a reduction or fracturing of gendered biolegitimacy through the interactions between men and providers in clinical settings. It is not the disease or threat of disease that constitutes the problem. I contend that men's decisions to delay or avoid care may be understood less as simply adhering to normative conceptions of masculinity and more about distancing themselves from medical interactions that render their masculinity and/or male identity as problematic and in need of intervention.

Threat and Compensation

That cancer is a threat to gender is a widely used narrative in activism, popular media, and the medical community itself. As sociologist Juanne Nancarrow Clarke argues, "the threat of [gender-specific cancer] seems to be less a threat to life itself than a threat to the proper, i.e., gendered, enactment of life" (2004, 549). Here, Clarke was specifically thinking through breast cancer in women and testicular cancer in men, but there is a different sort of threat at hand when men require treatment for breast or gynecological cancers. There is the possibility that, because these cancers are linked to body parts symbolic of femininity and womanhood, these cancers being diagnosed locates men in greater proximity to femininity, which then poses a threat to their masculinity. Another threat explained by men in this study was that the presence of men in spaces designated for women threatens the feminine underpinnings of the space and women patients. As a result, men and their providers engage in various practices to compensate for these threats.

Entering the Clinic

When men seek care for cancers deemed "female specific," they may begin with a primary care physician, but if more specialized interventions are needed they may find themselves in clinical spaces delineated for women. This can be a significant shift in treatment because the physical, visual, and interactional environment of these different spaces may be clearly influenced by normative ideas about femininity. Further, these different settings can have a specific feel that lets men know whether or not they belong.

Joe exclusively sought routine gynecological care through family medicine practices because he believed "family practitioners have a much better, warm view of trans people than internal medicine does. That's just the way I've always looked at it." Joe is making a distinction here between two primary care specialties: family medicine and internal medicine. Although physicians in these specialties receive similar types of training, internal medicine is centered more on inpatient hospital rather than outpatient clinic training. Even within primary care, there can be differences in how trans men expect to be seen. Joe's comment is an allusion to aligning internal medicine with more specialized types of medical care like gynecology. For Joe, family medicine is the type of primary care that is less beholden to normative ideologies of gender in favor of focusing on individual patients. According to Joe, as the care becomes more specialized, so too does the entrenchment of these ideologies in care.

When a man leaves the space of his primary care physician for more specialized care, one of the first indicators that he is entering a clearly gendered space is the title of the clinic. Often clinics and imaging centers have "women" somewhere in the name, and the logos for these spaces are also often clearly gendered. Joe described the logo of one clinic as a drawing of a "horrendous stick figure, lady, thing, with a really obviously pregnant belly and really prominent breasts." A Google search for "gynecology clinic logo" provides a plethora of examples of this type of imagery. Swirling script, soft colors (especially pink), images of flowers (forever linked to vaginas, as proven by Georgia O'Keefe), pregnant figures, and long-haired and breasted figures holding babies are the hallmarks of these logos. Joe went on to explain that the name, logo, and décor of a clinic were signs that he did not belong: "I recognized that I was going into an office that 99.99 percent of the time is used solely for cis women. I thought of it as enemy territory. . . . It helps to give yourself a little narrative, so I was going into enemy territory."

For Joe and some of the other trans men, thinking in these terms allowed them to brace themselves for the disruption that seeking care might mean for their identities. By entering spaces designated for women, trans men had to find ways to manage the delegitimizing effects that this care could produce specifically by virtue of how they were perceived by providers. The physical features of the space were an indicator of whether trans men would be perceived as men and/or as a problem for providers.

While trans men might reasonably expect to confront highly gendered spaces, cis men are not always so prepared, even after a breast cancer diagnosis. Tim, for example, was taken by surprise when he was sent to a women's clinic for a mammogram: "So, the [doctor] scheduled me for [a mammogram], and I went. I knew exactly the place he sent me. I walk in, and they said, 'It's the building behind you, not this. This is the MRI place.' So, I walk in [the other building], and the suite they're sending me to, it's a women's clinic." Simply the name of a clinic can give a man pause upon entering. Joe's and Tim's responses reflect what has come to be called the "therapeutic environment" in medical and cultural geography. This term includes everything from the clinical space (inclusive of the décor) to the sociocultural factors that merge together in the process of care (Gillespie 2002; Williams 2002).

Some trans men described therapeutic environments that were distinctly nongendered. The space where Erik received care is like a "hotel lobby . . .

stylistically it's nice . . . everything looks kind of new." Erik had only positive reactions to the care he received in this clinic and unequivocally felt like he belonged. He explained further:

> Here is a guy sitting in your waiting room in the OB/GYN clinic, and we're talking about a receptionist, right? Not a medical provider, not a nurse, like not a doctor, not a nurse [*sic*], this was a receptionist, and who knows what training this person has had, but the patient, who is a man, comes up, gives you the paperwork and says, "I'm here to see XYZ doctor." They were never confused as to why I was there. They never looked at me funny. They always looked me in the eye, and they treated me like every other person, you know?

For Erik, the physical space of the clinic reflected the way he felt he was perceived and treated by office staff and by clinicians. The initial interactions that Erik described are the first human contact within the therapeutic environment, and they are important ones. Both cis and trans men described situations in which checking in and waiting to meet providers felt fraught. Typically, the discomfort men described related to assumptions by clinical staff that patients were necessarily women. These assumptions were manifest in paperwork, verbal statements, and the structuring of where men could be in certain waiting rooms.

After adjusting to his initial surprise at being sent to a "women's clinic" for a mammogram, Tim described entering the waiting area: "I walk into the women's clinic, and they needed a clipboard [filled out with personal information]. The first two [questions] it was like, okay, have you been feeling well or sick or whatever. Then they started, like, 'When was your last menstrual cycle? Are you pregnant?'" The lack of inclusivity and gender neutrality on intake forms is something that trans men routinely dealt with. A common call to prevent this type of microaggression is to alter clinic policies and procedures to prevent these moments of invalidation. For example, intake forms might have an open space where patients can insert their preferred pronouns or gender identity, rather than having a choice of only male or female.

Where most trans men advocated for these kinds of changes to the intake forms due to their alienating impact, Ezra (a cis man with breast cancer) dismissed the importance of forms and was almost apologetic about his discomfort: "It's not a big deal. Most of the patients are women, so the forms ask you whether you're pregnant, you know. I mean, you could think of a form that doesn't, but, you know, I'm not going to insist that they invent one for me." The difference in how trans and cis men react to gender assumptions on intake forms reflects the degree to which these different groups of men can assume gendered biolegitimacy. For most of the cis men, there was no question that they were men in the space of the clinic. Providers might behave as if a patient's masculinity were threatened because he had breast cancer, but this was not typically combined with interactions that questioned a patient's status as a man.

Intake forms are not the only component of a patient's entrance into a therapeutic environment. As Erik's narrative indicated, interactions with front desk staff set a tone for the resulting clinical examination. Although many trans men expected to be misgendered, it was also a possibility for cis men. Larry, who received care at a well-respected cancer research facility with a large male patient population, expressed his frustration with women's clinics:

> It's a big issue. The breast center has a very nice big waiting room, and I can't tell you how many times I would be called "Mrs. Smith." One time I was there for an ultrasound to check the progress of the chemo, and I kept waiting and I kept waiting and I kept waiting, and it was like forty-five minutes past my appointment, and I went up to the desk, and I said, "I'd just like to know when I'm going to be called back," and she said, "Oh, well let me check—there's a delay because there are a lot of women back there, and they didn't want them to get all flustered." . . . After a mammogram, there's the main doors that you go in, and there's like a side door over at the far side, and several times they would direct me to go out that—like the back door, so to speak. Because you know the women are sitting in there in gowns in sort of the little waiting room to be called in. I mean you feel strange enough having what's perceived as a woman's disease.

Larry was referred to by the wrong gendered honorific, and his presence had to be managed by medical staff so as not to "fluster" the women patients who claimed the space of the clinic. Frequently, office staff even assumed that Larry was in the wrong place. When he stepped up to the window to register for a mammogram, "the person sitting behind there would say, 'Oh, you need to go to the third window' [for prostate screenings]." The need to minimize the impact of men in women's health care spaces was reiterated by many trans and cis men.

Larry's experience of awkward misgendering was shared by many trans men. For Zach, a trans man, the repetition of these experiences in a range of health care settings ultimately led to him avoiding cancer screenings: "I always looked like a guy, and I just had a girl's name. And so whenever I was in the doctor's office and my name would be called, it would be embarrassing for me to get up because people would be like, 'Oh, I thought that was a guy.' And so now when I'm finally, like, okay, I have a name that finally matches the way

I look, I'd rather not go back into a situation, like I did for eighteen years of my life, where I get called and I have to get up and it's awkward."

The fact that although many cis men explained that the care spaces they inhabited in order to receive a breast cancer diagnosis were distinctly gendered, it is notable that Larry was the only one who spoke at length about how this impacted his care. Most cisgender men have a lifetime of systemic gender capital and social privilege upon which they can draw in these situations, allowing them to minimize the affront of microaggressions in intake forms and from intake staff.[5] Generally, these interpersonal gaffs were understood by cis men as annoying and unpleasant, but fairly easy to move past.

As the only gay cis man in this study, Larry had a more contested degree of gender capital than that of the straight cis men. For Larry, the process of grappling with his sexuality and gender as a young man had left him extremely secure in his masculinity as an adult. As a result, his breast cancer diagnosis was unsettling, but it did not disrupt his sense of masculine identity. Larry shared, "Being a single gay male as I was at the time and had lived my adult life, you know, it has an added sort of twist to, oh, that's a woman's disease. . . . But in no way has it threatened my manhood . . . I don't remember a time in my life when I wasn't dealing with my sexuality. It's not like, oh, this makes me less of a man to have breast cancer." For Larry, coming to terms with his sexuality included grappling with his gender identity. "There were influences within the family that—I saw being feminine or being a woman was more ideal. And so I went through times when it was, like, questioning, you know, being—being male." Larry describes dealing with these aspects of identity as eventually allowing him to develop a sense of security in his masculinity, although he acknowledged that his way of being a man differed from hegemonic ideals.

Larry, like the many trans men participants, had spent a considerable amount of energy to cultivating a sense of stability in his sense of himself as a man. Over the course of Larry's life, he was able to reconcile the socially constructed connection between being gay and being feminine with his own version of masculinity. This process allowed him to understand himself as "a man dealing with a woman's disease" without questioning his masculinity. This work was protective against cancer being threatening, but it was not protective for managing the microaggressions of how he was perceived by others.

For Larry as a gay man and for the many trans men participants, their claims to gendered biolegitimacy have not always been supported by other people. It is the treatment of a person by others—particularly those with authority over the body—rather than any actual condition of health or the physical body that becomes significant in cultivating gendered biolegitimacy.

The Threat of Care

After navigating intake forms and waiting rooms, men face clinical exams and interactions with medical providers. It is during these interactions that the alignment between men's identities, bodies, standards of care, and provider expectations may come into conflict. Largely, cisgender men are afforded social recognition throughout medical interactions. That is, although there may be initial discomfort, cis men are seen as and treated by health care providers as men who need care, not as curiosities. Although men are not the expected breast cancer patient, they are conceivable to providers because their bodies and identities match. Their bodies do not need to change; rather, the medical interaction needs to change to ensure that treatment does not threaten the alignment between patient identity, body, and cultural expectations for gendered bodies.

Both trans and cis men have the wrong gender for the medical care they seek. In the case of cisgender men, the identities and bodies of the patients are aligned with what is normatively expected in a medical exam. They simply were unlucky to be diagnosed with a disease associated with women. In other words, the identities and bodies of cis men are aligned, and their bodies (because of the presence of a tumor) align with medical care. Their identities and care do not align, however, because breast cancer care is predicated on a standard of female-identified women. Within the context of the medical exam, the bodies of trans men are aligned with gynecological care, but their identities are not. Cis men essentially get the wrong cancer, and trans men have the wrong gender. Breast cancer care providers can accommodate the strangeness of men breast cancer patients because they see these men as victims of a disease that is outside of their control.

Trans men largely described their sense that, according to normative ideologies, their bodies and identities do not align and that, based on previous clinical experiences, this may create obstacles for care. Earlier in this chapter, I quoted Isaac's concern that medical providers can become incapable of treating him when they learn that he is not a cis man. Peter went a bit further in his explanation of this phenomenon. It is not necessarily that providers are incapable of treating trans men, but more that the care provided feels off to patients. He described seeking care in an emergency department:

> So I go in, and the stuff is pouring out of my vagina, I need some help. The person that I meet with is like, "I hear you. That is terrible. I also have a vagina." So we're on the same page. We're, like, going to deal with it. [And she tells me the] treatment options: you can have a cream that

> you shoot up into your vagina. You do it at night, and it's kind of going to leak out, you might want to wear a panty liner. And I'm thinking: in my boxer shorts? How? No. [And the other option is] you could take a pill that will also kill off other good flora and fauna in your system. So I tell her I'll take the pills. And she says, "Really? I'm shocked." That's what she said: "I'm shocked." I said, "Are you? Tell me about that." She said, "Well, were I making this choice for myself, I would totally go with the localized treatment because I know that it would treat only the bad stuff and it would be over in a week." And I said, "I totally hear you, but I'm trying to make the things stop pouring out of my body. I don't want to introduce more things that are going to come out, and I think it's hilarious that you would suggest a panty liner to me."

Peter's story reflects experiences of trans men in which providers can struggle to incorporate the realities of a patient's gender identity into the provider's assessment of appropriate care. Often providers do not intend to cause harm or discomfort for their patients. In Peter's case, his nurse was genuinely puzzled by his resistance to local treatment. Her confusion reflects the taken-for-granted assumption in medicine that gynecological patients share a common experience as women. Culturally and medically, gender is a binary system. Encountering a patient who troubles a binary understanding of gender or the relationship between bodies and gender identities requires the provider to undo a lifetime of exposure to cultural norms about femininity, masculinity, and the bodies associated with each.

The cultural link between the body parts examined in breast and gynecological care was clear to many men in this study. Erik spoke passionately about the ways in which certain organs are laden with meanings about sex, sexuality, and gender: "When it comes to something like gynecological care, we're talking about parts of people's bodies that are highly sexual. I mean, they're all kinds of things, right? They're highly arousable. They're highly sexual. They're highly sexualized. They're highly gendered." Despite this cultural understanding of the body, many trans men had different ways of thinking about their bodies, even when they understood that their providers might adhere to the culturally normative association explained by Erik. Joe, for example, saw no conflict between his body and his identity, other than in the context of obtaining gynecological care. In everyday life, Joe did not see his genitals as a source of anxiety.

> The exterior genitalia is [*sic*] very much associated with a gender I am not. I don't want anyone to judge my gender based on my genitalia. While I feel pretty secure in my gender, I think there is always that nagging voice

> from my head from when I was a kid, from when I was judged incorrectly on my gender based on my external features . . . there's a large part of me that's very much afraid that I would still be judged female by someone looking at my genitalia . . . I'm not a trans guy who feels like he needs a penis. I don't need a penis . . . I don't feel any sort of connection with the thought of having a penis. On the other hand . . . the uterus and the ovaries don't bug me either. They're inside, and I really don't care about them other than I would prefer they not give me cancer and kill me.

The overt attention to "purportedly gendered body parts" (Spade 2011) in gynecology links the body (internal reproductive organs and external genitalia) to a particular social category (female). As Joe indicates, his personal comfort with his body and identity are devalued within gynecological interactions. In this moment, Joe's body becomes a site of struggle between his identity, the institutional discourse of gynecology, and cultural norms of femininity.

To be certain, not all trans men recounted their gynecological exam experiences in this way. Jamie explained that his provider consistently tried to create a comfortable atmosphere where his body and identity were unproblematic: "I think, for me, the key was always feeling like my provider could understand that my gender was one thing, but my body was what it was. The fact that my gender was masculine didn't mean that they could ignore the female parts of my body." Several trans men felt that health care providers were able to respect both the identity and body of the patient in front of them. These statements affirm research findings that providers' use of appropriate pronouns and names is very influential in establishing comfort and trust in medical care for trans patients (Hagen and Galupo 2014). Erik was never made to feel like his identity and body were medically at odds.

> I present very masculinely. I do this on purpose. I'm not unaware of the fact that I'm saying to the world, like, "I want you to look at me like a man," you know? And they responded to what I felt like I was communicating on an unspoken level, and they never challenged that. They never questioned it. They just responded to Erik. They responded to my whole person rather than being like, oh, you're a trans person, and these are a collection of symptoms, or problems, or concerns, or you must have this problem because you're trans, or you must have this concern because you're trans, or you must have this kind of anatomy. They never assumed what my genitalia was, which also meant a lot to me . . . I got to live in a world where it was normal to be a guy with a vagina. Nobody was freaked out by that. Nobody had questions. Nobody didn't know how to treat

> me. . . . They treat me like a human. It's not weird or abnormal, or uncomfortable that I am a guy with a beard who has a vagina, you know?

Erik attributed his positive interactions with the medical profession to trust and communication. Taking Erik's identity and body at face value was critical to establishing a trusting environment for care. Erik speaks to the ways in which his medical providers were able to see his identity and his body as a unified whole, rather than as discordant and troubling. Jamie also explained that the staff and providers at the gynecology clinic where he received care "checked in with me about pronouns" and consistently made an effort to create a comfortable atmosphere where his body and identity were unproblematic. When staff and providers accept the gender presented by trans men and proceed with care in a way that minimizes the influence of gender ideologies in clinical interactions, they are actually working to reinforce men's gender biolegitimacy by making unremarkable the relationship between men's identities and bodies while avoiding judging these men based on normative ideologies of gender.

Some men described ways that providers behaved in ways clearly intended to bolster men's masculinity. Ezra's mammography technician assured him that "they do men all the time." Henry's technician provided reassurance by continually referring to the imaging as a "man-o-gram." When Larry went for his first mammogram, he was surprised and comforted by the efforts of the technician to make him feel at ease: "The technician was thoughtful enough to go dig in a cabinet for a tattered blue basic, little patterned gown like you get at the doctor's office instead of just pulling a pink gown from the stack that was out on the counter." Joe similarly mentioned that his gynecologist found him a "non-pink gown." These efforts are symbolic gestures indicating that the male-bodied patient was accepted in this generally women-specific space. However, they also signaled that these men were noticeably out of place and that by being in a space defined by femininity, the masculinity of these men might be threatened.

This presumed threat was often explained away by men. In a quote earlier in this chapter, Larry asserted that being gay protected him from breast cancer disrupting his sense of self because his sexuality distanced him from the pressures of hegemonic masculinity. Most of the straight cis men also minimized the potential for breast cancer to threaten their identities. Ted recognized that breast cancer might be threatening for some men, but not for him: "I think there really is an element for men that it's difficult to accept that you might have this disease that's always associated with women and rightfully so. And I think for probably most men that would make them feel at the very least uncomfortable.

I can't myself say that it has affected me that way . . . I've always been comfortable with who I am, and I certainly don't think of myself as particularly macho."

Adding specificity to claims of nonconformity to hegemonic masculinity, Ed talked about being smaller than average for a man and mentioned being an avid ballroom dancer, an activity not currently considered especially masculine, particularly for a white man (Craig 2014). According to Ed, these characteristics combined into an unconventional masculinity that protected him from feeling threatened as a man by his diagnosis. Ed, Larry, and Ted each framed their diagnosis around their understanding of themselves as atypical or non-macho men. Although they acknowledged that breast cancer could be problematic for other men, they felt protected from such threats because they situate themselves outside hegemonic norms.

The way that the men spoke about identity threats related to cancers commonly considered "female specific" tended to reject the idea that cancer or their body parts could threaten their masculinity or their legitimacy as men. Even if these men downplayed the gender threat of cancer, they remained acutely aware that they were out of place. Joe and Gabe were especially clear that trans men are out of place during gynecological care. Most of the trans men shared stories about being referred to by the wrong name or pronouns, having providers surprised when they entered the exam room, and having to answer questions that felt inappropriately invasive about their identities and unrelated to the care at hand.

While trans men's identities did not fit the space of the exam and thus called into question the legitimacy of their bodies, cis men described the physical sense of not fitting into the diagnostic machinery. While standing, a patient's breast is sandwiched between two plates. Tim vividly remembered the pain associated with mammograms: "If you're a svelte, small-breasted woman or a male it does kind of hurt. . . . The nurse adjusted the height [of the machine]. She winked and grabbed my nipple . . . and pulled as hard as she could . . . and then clamped it down." Men (and women whose bodies do not fulfill cultural ideals of appropriately breasted women) have difficulty fitting into mammogram machines. Henry laughed when asked about mammograms and said, "It's a pretty tight fit." Frank felt fortunate to have "some tissue there so they didn't have a hard time getting me onto the machine." Larry described in detail how the lack of tissue was addressed: "They start way around, almost like on your back. They sort of push around from under your arm and gather enough sort of whatever to put it in the machine. It was strange at first. I'm used to it now."

Lack of tissue is not the only complicating factor when men receive mammograms. The location of body hair led to a humorous first experience for James:

"The first one was rather hysterical. Because [laughs] I have a really hairy chest and I don't have large man boobs [laughs], okay? And when I was there for the mammogram, we get it into the device and crank it down, and it would pop out [laughs] because of the hair. And what would normally be like a five-minute ordeal for a woman turned into a twenty-minute thing for me."

Mammography machines are designed for easily accessible, hairless breasts. Given that mammograms are often conducted in women-centered clinics, everything from intake forms, to physically navigating the clinic, to the exam itself can be alienating for men. There are constant reminders that men's bodies are wrong for the space and care that these clinics provide. Ezra admitted to feeling "a little odd" and "a little weird" at the breast clinic. He believed that this was a common experience for men who "experience cultural dissonance when they go into this very female environment." It is important to note that cis men did not think that the clinics themselves should change, despite experiencing breast cancer care as relative outsiders.

I understand the tension created by men seeking care intended for women's bodies and predicated on assumptions about femininity through the concepts of masculine overcompensation and undercompensation (Young 2017). Masculine overcompensation explains the reaction of some men who meet threats to their masculinity with "compensatory increases in culturally masculine behavior" (2017, 1346). In the case of breast cancer care, cis men patients did not report masculine overcompensation. Rather, this theoretical lens fits the behaviors of the providers who use language, gown color, and other interactions to remind patients that they are, in fact, still men. Providers accustomed to treating cisgender women through feminized forms of interaction and treatment reportedly behaved in ways that align with masculine overcompensation to account for the presumed masculinity of men with breast cancer and sometimes for trans men in gynecological clinics. That is, the providers assumed a threat to masculinity and acted to bolster men against this perceived threat, whether or not the men felt threatened.

Because providers were doing the work of masculine overcompensation for their cis men patients and because cis men did not see their gender as threatened, cis men could engage in masculine undercompensation, where "archetypal masculinity is selectively tempered" (Young 2017, 1348). In so doing, they reinforced the idea of the clinic as a woman's space and women's (and femininity's) centrality in the cultural discourse on breast cancer as well as in medical interactions. This then adds to men's masculinity by placing individual men in alignment with ideals of chivalry and feminism. Such undercompensation is evident in cis men's statements that they do not want to have new forms made for them or their understanding of breast cancer clinics as properly women's spaces.

Trans men do not share this ability to respond to threats to their identities through masculine undercompensation. While cis men reported instances of providers assuring them through clinical interactions that they were unequivocally men, trans men more regularly explained that medical interactions worked to delegitimize their status as men. It is unclear whether similar masculine overcompensation on the part of providers would be uniformly welcomed by trans men. It is possible that trans men's history of previously being perceived as women may render them skeptical of the more overt displays of idealized masculinity (see Schilt 2010). While cis men tend to embrace normative masculinity in general, the interactions of trans men with the health care system suggest a degree of resistance to idealized masculine embodiment.

The ways the men explained their exam experiences suggest that the biggest threat to masculinity and male identity is not the possibility or reality of cancer in a body part gendered female. Instead it is how medical care for these cancers is predicated on assumptions about bodies and identities that do not fit the men in question. Additionally, the men in this study described their lack of fit with the norms of masculinity. This is an ideal example of "discursive distancing" (Bridges and Pascoe 2014). It is important to recognize that even when men create distance from hegemonic masculinity, as when the men in this study insisted that they are not "macho-man types," these hybrid masculinities are still "reiterating gendered relations of power and inequality" (Bridges and Pascoe 2014, 252). For cis men in particular, the potential threat of breast cancer as a feminizing experience could be alleviated by distancing themselves from hegemonic masculinity. At the same time, the men were quite clear about their interloper status in women's health care spaces and breast cancer activism. By distinguishing themselves from "typical" men, they were able to protect themselves from the potential for breast cancer to render them "not men" or "like women."

Women's Health and Activism

Ever conscious of being men in women's spaces, the men in this study were eager to clarify that they were not trying to diminish the historic and contemporary inequalities that women face in health care. In their desire to acknowledge the centrality of women to breast cancer care and activism, cis men described instances of affirming masculine power through a discourse of protecting women. This framing then granted the cis men the right of access to the feminized space of clinic and explained their behaviors once in that space (on the vulnerability of women and their supposed need for protection from the threat of masculinity, see Hollander 2001; Westbrook 2008; Westbrook and Schilt 2014).

The cis men I spoke with were very cautious about detracting from women's place at the center of breast cancer discourse. They were adamant that there was a need for greater awareness of breast cancer in men, but were cautious about causing any affront to women with breast cancer. Given his advocacy for men with breast cancer, Tim felt that this was a concern for breast cancer survivors.

> I'm not trying to take anything away from women. Sometimes, other breast cancer survivors kind of turn their nose. They're like, this is our thing. He's trying to steal our thunder. Absolutely not. I'm not trying to do any of that. I'm just trying to build the awareness that men can get it too. . . . If we can build the awareness and try to quit having men be so stubborn and go to the doctor when they feel that something is wrong and not waiting too long, that's what we're just trying to do. . . . We're trying to, you know, make it pink and blue.

In breast cancer culture, women and femininity are at the center. Larry describes it as "a sorority or a girls' club." This emphasis extends into the treatment centers, which are designed specifically for women. Although many of the men and women who participated in this project were unequivocally critical of Pink Ribbon activism, raising awareness remained an important concern for them. Regardless of the men's stance on the Pink Ribbon, they, like Tim, recognized the importance of preserving these spaces and breast cancer culture for women.

Whether or not men were familiar with the history of women's health activism, breast and gynecological cancer care were inherently linked to women. Trans men were somewhat more critical of the presumed femininity intrinsic to the design of health care facilities and the behavior of providers. Cis men tended to dismiss the ways that these ideologies shaped the spaces of care, but they wanted to increase awareness that men also could get breast cancer. These men had a more additive vision in which health care remained the same but included men. In contrast, trans men were more likely to think about changing the care to be more inclusive of all patients.

Conclusion

The contrasts in how trans and cis men described the ways in which their bodies and identities intersect in the context of breast and gynecological care produce a telling story about masculinity. Although both groups of men indicate that supposedly female body parts do not threaten their personal identity as men, the perceptions of and treatment by providers are shaped by, and thus reinforce, norms of masculinity. The narratives of the cis men indicated that they benefited in medical interactions because the providers perceived the bodies and identities of the cis men to be aligned with sociocultural imaginaries of male embodiment. As such, the stories relayed suggest that providers attempted to mitigate the possibility of breast cancer as threatening to men patients by bolstering their masculinity, thus reinforcing the power of normative ideas about gender in determining the legitimacy of bodies. For the trans men, this was never a certainty. Instead, trans men constantly ran the risk of their identities and bodies being questioned and deemed illegitimate by their providers because they voluntarily entered health care environments intended for women.

The stories in this chapter recount varying relationships between men's bodies, identities, masculinity, and femininity as understood within medical interactions. Although normative expectations of gendered embodiment link breasts, uteri, and ovaries with women/femininity, and penises and testicles with men/masculinity, the reality is that these relationships are much more ambiguous than many would like to believe. Although both trans men and cis men are marked as "wrong bodies" within female cancer care, the ways in which these bodies and identities are managed during medical interactions vary widely and produce a range of patient experiences. Cultural norms of masculinity become guides for cis men patients, trans men patients, and (especially) their providers while navigating breast and gynecological cancer treatment.

What the experiences told by men in this chapter make clear is the importance of visibility to medical interactions. Both trans and cis men relayed that it was important to be seen as men by their providers; trans men often felt overly visible to the point of feeling exposed. Whether or not men were seen as men, along with the degree to which their presence and visibility might make others uncomfortable, had an important impact on how these men experienced medical care.

In order for medical professionals to bolster men's biolegitimacy, the men must be visible. However, too much visibility can challenge normative expectations for gendered embodiment and lead to a belief that certain spaces or conditions will either disrupt the gender identity of patients or otherwise distress those around them. The subtleties of how clinical spaces are organized and how men are shepherded through these spaces highlight the degree to which normative expectations of gendered embodiment shape men's experiences of health care.

Chapter 2

Choosing Mastectomy

Breasts are a culturally significant marker of womanhood, and breast cancer is culturally understood not only as a major health risk but also as a threat to femininity. Whether breast cancer or BRCA has been diagnosed, cisgender women confront a series of decisions about what sort of medical interventions they should pursue, including the possibility of prophylactic bilateral (in the case of a BRCA diagnosis) or contralateral (in the case of a breast cancer diagnosis) mastectomy. In making these decisions, cis women may find themselves in tension with physicians and ideologies of gender. This chapter explores the choices of thirty-three women with breast cancer or BRCA mutations to pursue prophylactic mastectomies and the way they make sense of this choice in the context of gender expectations for female embodiment. The story of bilateral prophylactic or contralateral mastectomy told by participants is about balancing health risks and fear, embodied identity, and the perceptions of others. A woman's relationship to her breasts before the diagnosis, family relationships, and sexuality all contribute to this decision-making process.

When they have a breast cancer diagnosis or a positive BRCA test, cisgender women have the option to seek prophylactic mastectomies as part of their treatment, but this intervention is only recommended by physicians for those who have tested positive for BRCA. In this chapter, I explore how women make decisions about choosing bilateral mastectomy and offer some explanations for why this choice is so disruptive to medical professionals and worthy of media coverage and debate. I suggest that while women draw on several factors in making their decisions, the controversial elements of this decision hinge on the disruption of heterosexual desire via alternative embodiments. These different ways of embodying identity as a woman cause potential fractures in gendered biolegitimacy, thus rendering mastectomied bodies invisible, unintelligible, and undesirable.

A breast cancer or BRCA diagnosis creates space for women to consider what breasts mean and to make choices about what sort of body they want to have. As Karen, a participant with breast cancer, explained, "breasts are for breastfeeding, and they are for sexual pleasure, and they are for conforming to some sort of norm about what a woman's supposed to look like." Each of these functions may be disrupted by a breast cancer or BRCA diagnosis. Women described balancing the relationship between breasts, motherhood, sexuality, and femininity with very real fears about the impact of a diagnosis; this balance was central to how the women explained their decisions to pursue prophylactic mastectomies. As women participants made sense of their decision about bilateral mastectomy, the most important factor for all was to manage the fear and anxiety that breast cancer presented. However, the meaning of breasts as an embodiment of motherhood, sexuality, and femininity factored into women's decisions about bilateral mastectomy as well, which offers insights into why a seemingly individual decision might become a public controversy.

Women typically made their decisions in consultation with health care providers, family and friends, and social networks for breast cancer survivors or BRCA-positive people. The decision to seek prophylactic mastectomy may put cisgender women in conflict with health care providers, family members, and internalized cultural expectations. Having the support of providers, family, or friends was frequently mentioned by women as helpful in their decision-making. The narratives of the women who chose mastectomy highlight the ways in which breasts variously symbolize risk and certain aspects of what it means to be a woman both for personal identity and in the eyes of others. Further, the ways in which participants explained their decisions illustrate a balance between their desire to be healthy (and thus act as good biocitizens) and their understanding of themselves as women. The framework of gendered biolegitimacy aids in unraveling this tension between patient and provider understandings of risk and making sense of the differing perspectives on the meaning of breasts to gender identity.

All thirty-three women in this study chose to undergo prophylactic bilateral mastectomy. Thirteen participants had a BRCA diagnosis, and twenty had breast cancer. The women ranged in age from twenty-two to seventy; the women with breast cancer were at the older end of the spectrum at the time of interview. Most women participants were younger than forty-five at the time of the diagnosis. This is statistically normal for those who undergo testing for BRCA but is young for those with breast cancer. The median age at diagnosis for breast cancer in the United States in 2018 was sixty-two (Howlader et al. 2019). Importantly, the American Cancer Society recommends that women begin yearly mammograms at age forty-five (Oeffinger et al. 2015). Eleven of the women received a breast cancer diagnosis before age forty-five.

Overall, the stories expressed here are those of women who entered the cycle of breast cancer care at a relatively younger age than typical of the general population. Four participants—Ellen, Ashley, Suzy, and Judy—underwent the surgery because cancer was present in both breasts. Even for these women, however, mastectomy was not deemed necessary by their physicians. Of these four, only Ashley had primary cancers in both breasts. For the other three, cancer metastasized from one breast to the other. Themes of risk management and the meaning of breasts, both culturally and personally, ran through the stories that women told about choosing mastectomy. The participants also spoke candidly about their considerations of the people around them (including future intimate partners) and showed their decisions to be deeply individual yet embedded within their social networks.

Fear

At the heart of women's narratives about BRCA and breast cancer was the anxiety caused by the increased frequency of mammograms and other such early detection measures after diagnosis. Choosing a bilateral mastectomy meant an end to an annual cycle of worry for the women who participated in this study. As Fran, a retired scientist with a history of suspicious mammograms and a breast cancer diagnosis, explained, "It was just like I've had enough of this . . . I just wanted to get rid of the whole situation. I just don't want this worry all the time." For Fran, the yearly cycle of a suspicious mammogram followed by various additional tests had created a great deal of anxiety; a pragmatist, she ultimately decided that removing the breast tissue would remove the worry associated with annual mammograms of her remaining breast. Katie, a BRCA-positive participant, explained, "I had this real love/hate relationship with my breasts. I loved them, but I was afraid of them. I was afraid of what they could do. I was afraid of what was inside of them." Fran's and Katie's fears were echoed by all the women in this study. Women with a breast cancer diagnosis wondered whether lumpectomy, chemotherapy, or radiation would eradicate the entire tumor, whether chemotherapy or radiation would have long-term side effects, and whether the cancer would return or spread to the other breast. Both the women with breast cancer and those with positive BRCA tests worried that abnormal mammograms, combined with sometimes numerous rounds of follow-up tests, would create intense stress. These concerns cannot be resolved by current medical knowledge and thus were fundamental catalysts for the women who chose contralateral prophylactic mastectomies.

This logic is not, however, routinely accepted by medical professionals or popular media, even though elective prophylactic mastectomies rates have risen steadily for more than a decade and are in increasing demand as a preventive breast cancer measure (Grimmer et al. 2015; Hawley, Jagsi, and Marrow 2014; Tracy et al. 2013; Tuttle et al. 2007; Zeichner et al. 2014). This surgical technique is characterized by the removal of both healthy breasts (bilateral prophylactic mastectomy) or by the removal of the remaining healthy breast after a breast cancer diagnosis (contralateral prophylactic mastectomies). Part of the rise in prophylactic mastectomy rates is due to increased availability of genetic testing for BRCA mutations and a growing medical consensus that prophylactic mastectomy is an appropriate response to a positive BRCA test.

The reality of increased surveillance compared with the promise that breast removal would be adequate for women who with a breast cancer diagnosis can lead some women to choose prophylactic mastectomies. Colleen had a medically necessary unilateral mastectomy after a breast cancer diagnosis and decided to have a contralateral mastectomy after a period of living with one breast. She came to the decision to have the other breast removed after she had become "fed up with everything, everything about breast cancer, and everything about screening and everything about all the MRIs [magnetic resonance imaging] and scans and everything."[1] Contrary to the common belief that early detection is the best defense against breast cancer, both Fran and Colleen indicated that they found the measures invasive and anxiety provoking, and that ultimately they detracted from their overall quality of life. These two women are representative of the many women in this study who associated increased surveillance with ongoing emotional distress. Further, these screening methods are hotly debated in the news media because researchers differ on the efficacy of various technologies for early detection (Elmore et al. 2015; Kerlikowske et al. 2013). The women who chose bilateral mastectomy felt that the scientific uncertainty and emotional turmoil of the tests were more discomfiting than removing their breasts.

Other women expressed doubt that other breast cancer treatments would be effective over the long term. Suzy's doctors tried to talk her out of a mastectomy, arguing they could remove the tumor and rule out recurrence through radiation treatments. Suzy was uneasy with this approach. "It would have just been too stressful for me to wonder if it's all gone and is the radiation really killing it?" Concern about the efficacy of radiation or chemotherapy and subsequent side effects was widespread among study participants. For these women, mastectomies produced far less anxiety than a lumpectomy combined with radiation and/or chemotherapy. Linda wanted medical intervention to be as short term as possible. Speaking about her options of lumpectomy and radiation or a mastectomy, she said,

> I wanted to avoid it [radiation] at all costs, and [my surgeon] said, "If you have a mastectomy you won't have to have radiation." I actually had to go home and let it register and call her back and say, "Did I hear you correctly, that if I have a mastectomy, I won't have to have radiation?" And she said, "Yes," and I said, "Sign me up—it's going to be a double."

Rachel also expressed concern about the potential side effects of nonsurgical treatments, despite ultimately choosing to undergo chemotherapy. Samantha, too, worried about the future health consequences of radiation, including the possibility of developing other forms of cancer. She had a long family history of various cancers and wanted to ensure that her decisions about breast cancer did not impact the treatment of any future cancer.[2] When she did contract breast cancer a second time, she expressed relief that she had not previously undergone radiation treatment. In the first bout with breast cancer, she decided against radiation because "down the road I might need it, and you can't radiate the same area twice." She also expressed concern about chemotherapy because she'd "seen what hell it's done to people." Her overall approach to her first cancer was aggressively noninvasive. During the second occurrence, Samantha chose mastectomy to avoid radiation, although her qualms with radiation had less to do with side effects than with the logistical difficulties she faced in getting to the clinic for treatment on a regular basis.

Decisions about treatment can be complicated by a lack of certainty on the part of medical providers. In Alison's experience, the medical recommendations were not clear. She recalls that her breast surgeon "initially wasn't sure if a lumpectomy would be adequate." The range of medical options and the occasional difficulty in assessing the full extent of breast cancer can create what seems to patients to be considerable uncertainty about the most effective treatments. In this study, women with breast cancer tended to feel that a mastectomy, either unilateral or bilateral, was the surest means to prevent future risk of recurrence or a new diagnosis in the other breast.

Where the health benefits of prophylactic mastectomy are not always clear for women with breast cancer (a point I return to in chapter 4), a BRCA-positive diagnosis commonly leads to prophylactic bilateral mastectomy. For many BRCA-positive women, health statistics make prophylactic mastectomy a foregone conclusion. Women in the general American population have about a

12 percent lifetime risk of breast cancer (National Cancer Institute 2018). Studies vary as to the exact lifetime risk for women with BRCA mutations, but researchers have assessed the risk as being significantly higher than that of the general population. The National Cancer Institute reports that women with the BRCA1 mutation have a 55 to 65 percent lifetime risk of breast cancer and women with the BRCA2 mutation have a 45 to 56 percent risk (National Cancer Institute 2018; Chen and Parmigiani 2007).[3] Other studies have suggested even higher lifetime risks, ranging from 45 percent for women with BRCA2 (Antoniou et al. 2003) to 82 percent if the woman is of Ashkenazi Jewish heritage (King et al. 2003). In addition to BRCA, there are ranges of other genetic and medical conditions that increase a woman's risk for breast cancer and can influence her physician's surgical recommendations.

The women who were BRCA positive in this study had to first decide whether to undergo genetic testing. In many cases, the women who chose testing had family histories of breast cancer occurring in women at relatively young ages. Acquiring this genetic knowledge empowered some women. Emily explained, "The reason I wanted to know in the first place was [with BRCA] there's something you can do. . . . Once I found out that I was positive it was a question of do I want to go through regular [breast cancer] screenings every six months?" She anticipated abnormal mammography results and wondered, "If they see any tiny little thing that looks abnormal, they still have to investigate it. So at that point they would do a needle biopsy, and you would wait around and find out if you have cancer or not."[4] The option to have a bilateral mastectomy meant that she could proactively do something to reduce her breast cancer risk and avoid unnecessary stress in the future.

Rachel also described facing the possibility of increased surveillance. "My thought process was just based out of fear. I didn't want to have that worry of it coming back. I would constantly be obsessing over lumps." These sentiments were shared by the women with breast cancer. The difference between the two groups is that BRCA-positive women had an array of statistics supporting their fears, while the women with breast cancer grounded their decisions in their personal history. In an era of biocitizenship, generalizable statistics hold more value in the biomedical community while personal experience remains less convincing within the medical community. The acceptance of fear and anxiety among cis women positive for BRCA may be partially attributed to the way these emotions are deployed in advertising campaigns by developers of BRCA testing procedures (Hesse-Biber 2014). Medical professionals have, perhaps, gone too far in maximizing the importance of fear in a patient's consideration of treatment options after a BRCA diagnosis while minimizing the fears of women after a breast cancer diagnosis given the major advancements made in awareness, diagnosis, and treatment of breast cancer.

In choosing prophylactic mastectomies, women with breast cancer (in contrast to women diagnosed with BRCA) confront medical institutions and the gender structure by failing to conform to medical standards of care and by questioning the embodiment expected through norms of femininity. This failure to conform to medical and gender norms suggests that fear in this situation is a potential catalyst for changes in the status quo. Women's decisions to request prophylactic mastectomies and physicians' willingness (or lack thereof) to perform the procedure are wrapped up in a culture of cancer fear and cultural expectations of gender that do not necessarily align. The decision to undergo prophylactic mastectomy is not simply a story of fear, however. It also marks a moment of disruption between gender identity and embodiment. This disruption provides an opportunity for women (and anyone listening to their stories) to question what it means to be a woman, what it means to embody womanhood or femininity, and to reflect on the other meanings breasts have and roles that they play in daily life.

The Meaning of Breasts

Karen, a woman with breast cancer, concisely explained what she believed to be the meaning of breasts: "In my mind breasts are for breastfeeding, and they are for sexual pleasure, and they are for conforming to some sort of norm about what a woman's supposed to look like." Not all women who shared their stories agreed with Karen, but much of what she described was significant to participants. The way women felt about their breasts sometimes conformed to normative expectations and sometimes did not. Regardless, the experiences women had with respect to their breasts leading up to the diagnosis served as a foundation for making sense of the decision to pursue prophylactic mastectomies.

Personal Feelings about Life with Breasts

Prior to diagnosis, women in this study had somewhat differing views of their breasts. For some participants, a general dissatisfaction with their breasts contributed to their decision to pursue bilateral mastectomies. Others expressed intensely positive feelings, generally in relation to sexuality or to breastfeeding.

Maggie, a competitive athlete, never liked her breasts and considered them discordant with her identity as genderqueer.[5] As soon as she was diagnosed with cancer, Maggie knew that she wanted her breasts removed.

> The second they told me that there would be a surgical plan, I said, "Well then I'm going to do a bilateral mastectomy." And to be 100 percent honest I never really liked my boobs anyway. Never liked having boobs, and I had *boobs*. . . . [The] surgeons didn't question me at all. They were like, "Okay then, that's totally appropriate," and they moved on . . . I think that I had a relatively unique experience. I talk to other people, and the sheer number of people who tell me that there was resistance to doing the bilateral because the other breast is healthy. [My doctors] were clearly able to meet me where I was and respect me as the person that I presented myself to be.

What is significant here is Maggie's connection between embodiment and how she wishes to be seen. Maggie did not wish to conform to norms of female embodiment, nor did she identify as male. Instead, Maggie imagined an embodied state that was outside of generally accepted binary norms. This, in turn, shaped her decisions after being diagnoses with breast cancer.

Women frequently cited frustration at having large breasts as a motivating factor in deciding to have bilateral mastectomy. Linda, for example, had considered breast reduction prior to mastectomy: "I was extremely large-breasted before this [laughs]. You're going to think I'm lying, but the thing is I was wearing a 40M bra, as in Mary, and falling out of it. I had girls everywhere . . . I hated these huge breasts. I have looked at reduction, I thought about reduction every single solitary day of my life." Large breasts were described by participants as limiting many aspects of everyday life, from the type of activities a woman could comfortably pursue to the kinds of clothes she could wear. Jody had also considered breast reduction before the positive BRCA diagnosis, saying "[I had] never really been happy with my breasts." Sally, also BRCA positive, described the difficulty of having breasts in her pursuits as a high school and college athlete: "[my breasts] were just too big for me, for my frame. They got in my way."

Aside from size, the appearance of prediagnosis breasts was distressing for some women. Judy described a painful adolescence and young adulthood marred by extremely large and lopsided breasts that grew at different rates.

> When I started going through puberty, my breasts were not growing at the same rate. And every woman's breasts are slightly different in size, okay? None of us have perfectly spherical symmetric breasts. Mine, however, was the difference between probably a 42C versus a 38B type thing. There was at least a two-size difference. . . . Gym class was torture. High

> school gym class back in the '70s when you all had to take showers together. Every other girl in the locker room has got these perky little cute boobs. I used to take my towel into the shower with me and open it up and kind of, you know—sort of like you're just standing there with your towel half-mast, so to speak. You're blocking everyone else's view, but you actually get the spray coming down on the front of you. Yet, you know, your towel's not getting wet, but nobody else can see you. But then somehow or another somebody found out, and then it spread like wildfire through the school. So I wouldn't get directly teased by it, but there was a certain group of boys that every time one of them went by they—went down the hallway past me or something—they would make a noise loud enough for everybody else to hear. And everybody that knew what that noise was knew that it was about me. So that was extremely humiliating.

Although large breasts are portrayed in popular culture as aesthetically pleasing and desirable, in the everyday lives of women they are often frustrating. As Judy's story shows, not only breast size but also the shape and symmetry of breasts are of great importance. For Judy, the way she was seen and treated by others led to a very distressing adolescence.

To be sure, not all the participants were unhappy with their breasts before their breast cancer or BRCA diagnosis, and many women had a strong connection to their breasts, as will become evident in the following sections. However, the previous comments provide a counternarrative to the predominant assumptions that big breasts are good and that no woman would possibly choose to remove her breasts if an alternative were possible. The relationship of breasts to gendered biolegitimacy is not uniform, and a woman's experience of being a person with breasts can influence the decisions she makes after a breast cancer or BRCA diagnosis.

Motherhood and Parenting

Parenting was a major factor in women's deliberations about prophylactic mastectomy. Participants discussed their experiences as parents, their potential desire to become parents, and the symbolism of breasts to motherhood. For some participants, their roles as parents were deeply connected to their fears about future incidences of breast cancer. Rachel was explicit about this: "When I was diagnosed [with breast cancer] I chose to have a mastectomy over a lumpectomy because I was [in my thirties], I still had young children, I was very afraid." Kate stated, "It goes back to the cancer equals death; I don't want to die. I need to get the cancer out of my body. I had two young children at the time. I was very focused on, you know, wanting to live as long as possible . . . I would like to live, and I would like to have my children under my care." The fear for these women was chiefly about staying alive for their children and being physically able to care for them.

This concern also played into the decisions of young women who did not have children at the time of their breast cancer or BRCA diagnosis. Colleen's knowledge that she wanted to have children and her oncologist's support were crucial in her decision to have a bilateral mastectomy.

> The new oncologist I was referred to was a woman, and I feel like she was maybe a little more sympathetic than the men I had seen. She actually brought mastectomy up when I met with her for the first time. She was, like, "If I was in your position I would do it in a heartbeat." She said, "Well you just got married, you can think about it now or you can think about doing it after you have children." That was like, oh wow, ok. I didn't really think about the timing for the kids, and yeah if I want to have kids, well, I don't want to do it after I have kids. First of all, another two more years that I have to worry, second of all, I'm going to have this major surgery with, you know, a kid or two running around? That felt horrible, so my decision was, all right, I want to do it, and let's do it now. I want to get this out of the way. I want to just go on with my life, then I can think about having kids.

Explicit in Colleen's statement is her concern about parenting young children while recovering from surgery. Although with her particular type of cancer mastectomy was a choice, the potential of recurrence and eventual surgery prompted her to choose the medical intervention she felt gave her the best chance for the future life she envisioned for herself.

The fear of not being around to care for one's children was also a strong motivator for women with BRCA. After growing up and watching several generations of women in her family die from breast cancer, Katie strongly believed that she "did not want another woman raising my children" and that she "wanted my children to see that a woman in her family could grow old. . . . It really felt like, knowing the fear I had lived with, I didn't want my children to live with that fear." For Michelle, the desire to have children and a long life in which to parent them directly influenced her decisions about surgery. After receiving her BRCA result, Michelle made a quick decision: "I kind of decided right then and there, going to have the mastectomy, no questions asked, sooner than later . . . I want to have kids; I want to have a family someday. I can have kids and I can do all the things I want to do without my boobs."

As women considered their role as parents, breasts symbolized a threat to their ability to parent. Yet in both the biomedical and sociocultural imaginary breasts symbolize motherhood through the act of breastfeeding. Although Michelle asserted that she could do all the things she wanted without boobs, women who wish to breastfeed lose that possibility with mastectomy.

For many women, breastfeeding was a deeply important experience. Karen was particularly forthright about the significance of breasts to parenting because of her ability to breastfeed: "I thought [my breasts] were fantastic. I thought they were just amazing [laughs]. They were, like, kind of magical [because they could instantly soothe my children]." Karen's positive feelings about breastfeeding allowed her to choose mastectomy because she had had such a positive experience breastfeeding and felt that her breasts had served a purpose. Because Karen was planning no future pregnancies, having a breasted body felt less important. For Fran, breastfeeding and her decision prior to diagnosis not to have more children similarly figured critically in her decision regarding mastectomy: "In fact, I'm sure that if I had been younger and had been planning on having another child, then I would not have had the mastectomy. . . . It's a great pleasure to feed a child with your breast. It's an extraordinary pleasure, and one knows that it's good for the child. On both of those accounts I would've done what I could to save the breast if I'd been planning on another child."

Liz also did not plan to have more children at the time of her breast cancer diagnosis. A positive experience breastfeeding her second child was significant in her decision to pursue bilateral mastectomy. Her first attempt at breastfeeding her oldest child had been painful and unsuccessful. With her second child, Liz breastfed with ease and remembered the time leading up to her mastectomy. She said, "I remember a couple nights waking up holding my breasts, and I feel like that was more of me saying goodbye and thank you, but it didn't really make me stop. I knew I was done having kids, so I felt like they had served their purpose in my life . . . I never saw my identity in my breasts, so I never felt that that piece of it—it was they served their purpose as me—for me as a mom, and I don't need them anymore." For Liz and Fran, breasts were important tools in early experiences of parenting, but were not tied to their personal identity or to their relationships with their children at the time of mastectomy.

Although the positive experience of breastfeeding enabled many women to let go of their breasts, it caused sadness in others. For Karen, breastfeeding was a particularly special bond with her youngest son: "Whenever people would [ask], how are you feeling about surgery coming up or whatever, I could be, like, oh, you know what, I'm okay with it . . . I mean I did some minimizing of it, like, whatever, my breast betrayed me, let's get rid of it; the other one's guilty by association, so, you know, begone with them. But if somebody asked me something around, like, the breastfeeding issue or anything, then that was like a trigger for tears, and—yeah, a lot of tears." Although conversations about breastfeeding caused pain for Karen, she still decided to have bilateral mastectomies because doing so was, in her opinion, the best option to ensure that she would be present and able to care for her children.

The fact that breastfeeding was mentioned so often during interviews fits broader U.S. trends concerning the importance of breastfeeding. In 2006, the American Academy of Pediatrics (AAP) and the American College of Obstetricians and Gynecologists (ACOG) jointly published the *Breastfeeding Handbook for Physicians* in response to the research finding that "only 71% of women ever start breastfeeding" (ACOG 2006). The U.S. Department of Health and Human Services also launched a campaign at that time to increase the incidence of women breastfeeding to 75 percent and to increase rates of prolonged breastfeeding (past six months) to 50 percent (ACOG 2006). The AAP released an updated policy statement on breastfeeding in which they argued that "breastfeeding and human milk are the normative standards for infant feeding and nutrition" (2012). The policy statement goes on to identify disparities in breastfeeding utilization and the benefits of breastfeeding to mothers and children. The policy ends with a recommendation that mothers exclusively breastfeed their children for six months, and continue to do so, along with introducing solids, for at least one year.

Following these statements, the AAP indicated various clinical practices that should be encouraged by physicians to promote breastfeeding. As a result of these efforts and those of breastfeeding advocacy groups such as the La Leche League, breastfeeding has achieved a strong cultural presence in the United States, despite the many controversies over public breastfeeding (Wallace 2014). Issues of visibility aside, breastfeeding is framed as an essential experience for both mother and child. To be a good mother is to breastfeed, according to the messaging now prevalent in U.S. society.

For women diagnosed with BRCA, the potential inability to participate in this purportedly magical and healthful experience presented difficulties for their decision-making, but it did not prevent women from choosing to have surgery. Emily characterized this dilemma as containing "a lot of emotional attachment involved in that [decision] because it's a rite of passage as a mother" and went on to remember being a small child when her mother received a breast cancer diagnosis: "I was envisioning myself potentially having a child who is one, two, three years old then potentially getting breast cancer. And I just couldn't justify that in my head, the possibility of having children and then potentially getting sick and dying [laughs]. I would rather—much rather, you know, forego the cosmetic—the cosmetic issues that are involved in having a mastectomy, and, you know, not be able to breastfeed but then be there for my children and see them grow up. So, you know, I'd rather live."

Michelle also felt sadness at the idea of losing the ability to breastfeed. At the time of our interview, several of her friends were pregnant or new moms, and they often discussed breastfeeding and pumping. Although Michelle told me that this "sounds like a huge pain in the ass," she also felt sadness. "I'm kind of sad I'm not going to be able to do it. It seems like a really great special bonding time with your baby, and nutritionally you pass so many good things on to your baby." She went on to say, "I know there are tons of people that are—that don't breastfeed, and their babies grow up beautifully and healthy, and they do have bonding time and all this stuff. So it's probably, you know, it's going to be fine that I'm not going to be able to do it, but it does kind of bum me out a little bit that I never even get to experience, and I feel like that's just a, a maternal thing. A special bonding maternal thing that I'm not going to get to experience."

The sense that breasts had fulfilled their purpose in sustaining the life of infants allowed some women to let them go; for other women, the connection to children made a mastectomy decision somewhat more difficult, particularly if they had not yet had children but planned to in the future. The importance of breastfeeding to women participants in this study reflects the current cultural landscape in which we live. Breastfeeding is largely considered healthy for both babies and people who give birth. Although the participants had to reconcile the meaning of bilateral mastectomy with the meaning they associated with breastfeeding, breast cancer and BRCA diagnoses gave a new primary meaning to breasts as threatening and fearsome. For those who were planning to have children, they needed to process what it would mean to have bilateral mastectomy and not breastfeed. For those who already had breastfed, the experience helped to provide a sense of closure around the function of breasts, thus allowing them to choose to remove their breasts.

Identity and Sexuality

Although women participants in this study could have mastectomies and still mother children, they found the question of what removing breasts meant for gender identity and sexuality more complicated. Breasts, particularly large breasts, are one of the most visible and representative features of womanhood and female sexuality. In the popular imagination, women are rarely portrayed as sexy without their breasts being somehow visible or identifiable. The unproblematic association between breasts, female identity, and sexuality was not uniformly accepted by the participants. Instead, the experience of bilateral mastectomy they described shows how this association is the end result of a process in which the primary way women can achieve gendered biolegitimacy is through heterosexual desirability. By choosing bilateral mastectomies, the women in this study offered a different way of imagining female embodiment and sexuality, one that exists outside the status quo. In other words, the work of achieving gendered biolegitimacy becomes evident as the participants describe their bodies, identities, and sexualities in relation to mastectomy.

A key contributor to women's concerns about their partners was sexuality. For many women, their breasts were integral to sexual intimacy. The women were often candid about the personal importance of their breasts for sexual pleasure. As Karen explained,

> I mean, it's a sexual organ that you don't have any more. You just lost a major erogenous zone, which is weird . . . I mean of course it would be a much bigger problem, in a practical sense, if you lost an arm or a leg, but it is still a body part that serves a certain function and that function is no longer there. I mean, you regain some feeling in the chest, but it's not the same kind of feeling obviously [laughs]. And it's also not complete; I mean there's still like a band right across the scar, that's basically numb. So that is weird.

The loss of this sexual function was upsetting for many women, although they considered it a worthwhile sacrifice with their concerns about future health risks. Still, feeling sexy and engaging in sexual acts proved difficult for some women both before and after surgery.

Karen's struggles with intimacy began before her surgery. She initially intended to have a single mastectomy because of the sexual importance she attributed to her breasts. This feeling changed in the time after her diagnosis.

> Every time my husband touched my breasts I would cry. Our entire relationship became breastless before I lost the breasts, so it was like, whatever, six or seven months of intimacy that didn't include them because that would take me out of the moment and make me cry. I'm, like, it would have been better if we could have like bound them up and put them away so that we could enjoy ourselves. So it became a much easier decision. Initially I wanted to keep the other breast, I'd say, primarily for sex. By the time I made it through all that other stuff, it was, like, you know what? It is just not that important as I thought it was.

Being touched after mastectomy was difficult for many women. After her bilateral mastectomy for BRCA, Michelle lamented the impact on her sexuality:

> Intimately it sucks. Like, it's totally lame. I used to have sensitive boobs. I don't like when people touch my chest at all now. I think a guy kind of gets the point after a few dates when I'm, like, don't touch my chest, or something. Or we'll make out or something, but I insist on leaving my bra on; I will not take my bra off. I think a guy kind of gets the point. And so, inevitably, you know, after four, five, six dates, whatever it is, it comes up.

The physical changes brought about by mastectomy are undoubtedly important to individual's intimate relationships. Given the importance of heterosexuality to the gender order at large, these individual struggles with sexuality indicate a greater cultural significance to the recent trends toward bilateral mastectomies. The choice to remove one's breasts alters the symbolic meaning of heterosexuality to the gender system because heterosexual desire is "the basis of the *difference between and complementarity of* femininity and masculinity" (Schippers 2007, 91, emphasis in original). As Fran's son explained, when she removed her breasts, she became a boy and a girl. That is, bilateral mastectomy took away the difference and complementarity that is produced by and integral to heterosexual desire and is fundamental to a gender system based on hierarchical relationships.

Although some women considered the sexual impact of surgery well in advance, Liz reported being particularly surprised by her sexual reaction: "I had not considered the sexual aspect of it; I hadn't considered that I would be self-conscious about it. That took me by surprise [laughs] because I just had never identified with my breasts and then, all of a sudden, I was self-conscious about it, and I was, like, why am I self-conscious about it?" For Liz, being touched meant that she could not ignore her experience with cancer. Every time her husband touched her chest, it was a reminder of what she had gone through and brought up her concerns about how her husband felt about her body. None of the women in this study expressed any regret about their decision to have bilateral mastectomy, yet their commitment to this choice did not make the impact on their sexuality any easier to handle. Sexiness is thus partially defined by a woman's sense of how her body looks both to herself and to her partner. Perhaps more important, however, is the role of touch in relation to breasts. Prior to surgery, the sensation of touch could be emotionally painful, even if the physical sensation was not. After surgery, women lost physical sensation and had to cope with what that meant for their experience of physical intimacy.

Several women also expressed concerns about their male partner's reactions to the loss of breasts, even though nearly every woman described her male partner as extremely supportive of her mastectomy decision. Many women mentioned that their male partners had eroticized their breasts. Ellen's concerns were compounded by her recent hysterectomy:

> My main concern through all this was, like, I didn't want to be like [my husband's] making love to another man. I had a hysterectomy a year after the mastectomies which put me in a sexual quandary. I didn't know if I was a man—am I a man, am I a woman, what am I? I don't know what I am. I was questioning who I was because I had no female parts anymore. And no desire for sex, either.

Losing her breasts, uterus, and ovaries significantly impacted Ellen's gender identity and her interest in sex. She had always liked her breasts and described them as "cute and perky." Her breasts were an important part of her identity, and losing them along with other parts that she linked to her gender identity and sexuality caused her to question how her husband perceived her. This is not unlike the experiences reported by women who have had hysterectomies, for whom "the ability to feel sexually attractive is an important component of self-identification for many contemporary women, as is the ability to feel sexual desire and erotic pleasure" (Elson 2004, 123–124).

Ellen's statement raises issues of gender identity and sexuality alongside the issue of sexual function. When Ellen questions her identity, she implies that this identity is a combination of gender and heterosexuality. Without the parts that make her female, her sexuality no longer makes sense in relation to her male husband. The relationality of both gender and sexuality are clear in her statements. When her gender is no longer obviously female to her, then the heterosexuality of both partners becomes questionable. Typically, a man's heterosexuality may be socially questioned because of his behaviors—his failure to "do masculinity." Ellen's experience suggests a deeper relational context in which a heterosexual man's identity can become questionable through his partnership with a woman who chooses to live flat and thus fails to "do femininity."

In addition to the impact on personal sexuality and the relationship with an intimate partner, Ellen's sexual quandary expresses the ways in which a person's sense of being a man or being a woman can be challenged by physical changes. Commonly held notions of gender identity include a sense that we each have a core gender identity. This is the logic underlying the "wrong body" narrative of transgender people. Ellen's story suggests that instead of a core gender identity that is unalterable, one's gender identity can be linked to secondary sex characteristics. Ellen questioned who she was because she had no female parts. Ellen's experience is almost the inverse of the mainstream transgender narrative. The visibility of gender matters not only for social interactions but also for personal identity.

Although losing one's breasts does not necessarily obstruct sexual interest, it can be difficult for many women to "feel sexy" after bilateral mastectomy. Maggie attributed this to her own reaction to surgery rather than to her wife's: "I think I feel more damaged than she sees me, just because of the scars. I have a hard time feeling sexy. I'm working on it [laughs]." Maggie's wife participated in all the decision-making surrounding Maggie's breast cancer diagnosis and remained consistently supportive. Despite this type of support from their partners, many women remained worried about how to appear sexy to them. Nicole's main concern about mastectomy was "feeling like I wasn't sexually attractive to my husband." Even though he tried to reassure her, Nicole felt that "I still want to be sexy in his eyes. I want the sexual attraction to still be there."

Catherine actively dealt with her concerns about being sexy by deciding to remain nude at all times while at home to help her husband become comfortable with her scars.

> I really do think my body is badass, but it's been hard to settle into the changes. My husband was really having a hard time, and I just decided, without even really telling him, that I was going to be nude around the house as often as possible. And it really helped me to see the beauty of my person, and I believe it helped him to accept the changes. . . . My thing is, how do we make this beautiful? I would love to see a bustier that just comes slightly out and away from the body and sort of just gives a little gentle peek of the scars. Like there is nothing to hide here. It's only beautiful. Unless of course we decide to buy into the idea that we are our breasts. And I can't be my breasts anymore because my breasts had to go [laughs]. So I don't want to. I want to figure out a way to make this sexy, desirable.

Catherine's association of beauty with sexiness points to a tendency among women who choose mastectomies to attend to their own aesthetic sensibilities. Although Catherine's decision to be nude as often as possible was partially for the benefit of her husband, she was also deeply concerned with her own impression of the beauty of her body. As with Maggie, what is at stake here is a woman's ability to see her body as beautiful or sexy after a mastectomy. Sexiness is not limited to a woman's self-image, however. According to participants, the impact on intimate partners, combined with a woman's sense of her own sexiness, were both important considerations as women navigated their self-image after choosing bilateral mastectomy.

In order to achieve gendered biolegitimacy, sexuality can play a role in legitimizing or delegitimizing bodies in relation to ideologies of gender. However, the importance of how others perceive us extends beyond the sexual sphere. To imagine new possibilities requires disruption of some kind: access to technologies of the body, and support from people close to you who also will support these body technologies.

Support Systems

Nearly all participants recounted receiving strong support from intimate partners, children, and other people close to them. Although participants emphasized the individual and personal nature of decisions about mastectomy, they also routinely talked about the importance of family and friends in helping them come to terms with the decision and its resulting physical changes.

Reactions of Partners

Most participants described the reactions of their spouses and partners as supportive. Alyssa told me that her husband "lost both of his parents when he was young, so he was absolutely terrified that he was also going to lose his wife." Consequently, he encouraged Alyssa to have a bilateral mastectomy. Similarly, Karen's husband told her that "any risk at all" was unacceptable and supported her decision to have a bilateral mastectomy. Here, partners are reflecting the kind of fear of mortality that many participants felt themselves upon receiving their diagnosis. The threat of death connected to breast cancer was strong enough for them that any measure seemed worthwhile, given that such interventions will reduce the potential for death.

This fear of death is unsurprising. Mortality rates for breast cancer have been declining since the 1990s, but the rate has been slowing since 2017 (American Cancer Society 2019). The story that sticks in the imagination is the statistics showing that for women cancer is the second leading cause of death after heart disease (Centers for Disease Control and Prevention 2019). The death rates from breast cancer are higher than all other cancers besides lung cancer (Breastcancer.org 2019). Death seems a very real outcome to women with breast cancer, and for their loved ones the fear of losing their partner seems more significant than concern over losing a partner's breasts.

For some spouses and significant others, watching their loved one experience the anxiety of medical testing led to them supporting mastectomy. The partners were again reflecting the concerns expressed by the women themselves about their anxiety over increased surveillance if they chose not to have bilateral mastectomies. Edie noted that everyone in her life was "supportive for the same reason, that they had seen how much anxiety it caused me for so long." Her husband "ultimately really realized how much anxiety [another breast cancer diagnosis] caused me, and so he's been very supportive." Colleen's husband also responded to her anxiety regarding a future recurrence. Although he was initially cautious about the idea, Colleen maintains that "ultimately he really recognized how much anxiety it caused me, and so he's been very supportive" even though he "probably had a little more hesitation than I did." Ellen described her husband as uniformly supportive. She remembered his response as "Whatever we have to do we're going to do. . . . You're my wife. I love you, and boobs aren't going to make a difference." This was the fairly standard response that women reported from their intimate partners.

Despite the unwavering support of their intimate partners, many women remained apprehensive about how their scars would impact their partner and their own sense of sexuality. Several women reported that their breasts were their intimate partner's favorite body part. Samantha was very careful to gauge her husband's comfort level:

> I think it also helped a lot that we talked about it beforehand—how he might feel, and afterwards showing him the scars—showing him the bandage and then the scar and asking him—watching his face and asking him, "How do you feel about this? And how do you feel about me having the other side off?" And, after surgery, he saw the bandage. And he looked very calm, and he said, "I'm okay with it. Are you in pain? Are you okay?"

Ultimately, Samantha's husband main concern was with her comfort and happiness. According to Samantha, "You couldn't ask for better than that." Their openness in discussing the changes in her body has, in her opinion, strengthened their relationship: "It's opened him up, which in a way makes me feel even stronger towards him if that makes any sense. He's showing that he's baring that more vulnerable—what we sometimes term as a vulnerable side to us, exposing our deepest thoughts. He's growing more and more comfortable with that."

Several women described a shift to greater emotional intimacy with their partners, which helped some women integrate their new, breastless bodies into their sense of themselves and into their relationship, and built up the gendered biolegitimacy of their new embodiment. Yet even when spouses were supportive, the physical changes sometimes remained difficult to navigate. Judy felt that her husband struggled deeply with her scars. She reported that although he initially indicated to her that he did not want to see her chest, eventually Judy decided that it was important that he saw. "I pulled my shirt up, and he goes, 'Oh my God, don't show me that again.' He's never seen them since." Because Judy didn't want to talk about it further, it was unclear in our interview what she felt was the source of her husband's discomfort.

Like breasts, scars can have many meanings. Rarely are scars seen as beautiful.[6] Aside from these normative cultural ideals, scars are also a very visible reminder of the threat of cancer, the risk of death, and the pain that a partner may have experienced. This can be hard for a loved one to take. The silence surrounding scars was, however, not just an individual issue with Judy's husband—ours is a culture in which scars should be covered up. We expect scars to be treated with various products to reduce their appearance or otherwise be made invisible. The visibility of scars and their impact on interactions was important to many participants in this research, including the men with breast cancer. This is a point to which I return in the next chapter.

Reactions of Children

Their relationships with their children and grandchildren were significant for these women as they chose mastectomy and then became accustomed to life after, particularly when living flat. Interactions with children required the women to explain their bodies and to confront the ways in which their bodies challenged cultural expectations of womanhood. In general, the women had a fairly matter-of-fact approach to explaining mastectomy and surgery. Ellen's grandchildren began calling her "Grandma Booby" after she "got [her] boobs cut off." Her youngest grandchild, who was an infant at the time of surgery, later asked her, "Well, why don't you have boobies?" Ellen responded, "Because they got sick, and the doctor had to take them away."

Ellen's simple and straightforward approach to explaining mastectomy was mirrored by how the women felt their children responded to their surgeries. Kate explained, "I'm the only body that my daughters know. This is it. I mean this is who I am. I haven't moved into any category that would be, like, 'Oh mom, your body is embarrassing because of breast cancer.'" Kate's now-teenage daughters grew up while their mother was having a mastectomy and complications from reconstruction. Now that she lives flat, she feels that her breasts are a nonissue with her kids.

Children can also help normalize a woman's body after surgery. Judy had an open-door policy with her son where he could come into her room under any circumstances. A few weeks after her mastectomies, her son came into her room while she was undressing.

> [My son] came in, and I said, "Stop!" And he goes, "What?" And I said, "I'm ready to pull my shirt above my head and put my pajamas on." And he comes in the rest of the way, and he says, "Okay, so?" And I said, "Well, you're going to see scars if you don't turn around." He goes, "Well, I don't care. Scars are scars." All right, so I flip my top up, and I turn towards him and he goes, "Yeah, what of it? They're scars." Okay. Put my pajamas on and said, "All right, what else did you want?" and we had an entire conversation afterwards. Never blinked an eye. Never batted, flinched, nothing, whereas my husband about puked.

While Judy's husband struggled with her recovering body, her son acted as if everything was fine. Likewise, Fran's son was immediately very supportive of her mastectomies and decision to remain flat. According to Fran, "he's really great. He said, 'So Mom, you'll be kind of like a minotaur. You'll be, like, girl on the bottom, boy on top.'" While not every woman would be pleased to be characterized as a mythological creature, Fran understood her son's comment to be one of acceptance and unquestioning support for what she intended to do.

The comment of Fran's son that she'd be both a girl and a boy is crucial to understanding some of the tension underlying prophylactic mastectomies. Breast cancer is culturally understood as a threat to a woman's health and life, and also to femininity more generally. Cancer threatens individual femininity by occurring in a body part deeply connected to motherhood and sexuality, both of which are intrinsically tied to normative femininity. Breast cancer threatens femininity on a cultural level. As a society, we invest vast sums of money in breast cancer research in order to "Save the Ta Tas." Clearly, breasts are of national cultural concern, not simply of interest to individual women. Mixing boy and girl, masculinity and femininity, in a single body is uncomfortable culturally.

Given that gender is culturally defined relationally as male and female, masculine and feminine are placed in opposition (see Connell 1987). Troubling this separation can create social anxieties (see Westbrook and Schilt 2014 on gender panics). The emphasis on saving breasts through increased awareness of breast cancer and the importance of regular screenings, as well as on the biomedical insistence that lumpectomies and radiation are just as good as mastectomies for treating cancer, lends a certain sacredness to breasts that is embedded in cultural ideals of what a woman's body should be. In addition, when cisgender women blur the bodily lines between man and woman by altering their bodies through mastectomy, they inadvertently call into question the assumption "that there are certain bodies, behaviors, personality traits, and desires that neatly match up to one or the other [gender] category" (Schippers 2007, 89–90).

The issue of authenticity and comfort also permeated Sally's understanding of her daughter's reaction to her bilateral mastectomy. Sally described her previously large breasts as negatively impacting her happiness. Now, she says that her daughter "sees me being happy because I don't have these giant boobs. She sees me being able to be more free in activities and just at home playing with her." Although breasts can be important to a woman's identity, they can also get in the way. For Sally, it was more important that her daughter see a woman moving freely in the world than to see her mother with breasts. The physical constraints placed on women are a cornerstone of feminist theories of the body (see, for example, Young 1980, 2005). Many of the women I interviewed believed in feminist ideals of empowerment; physical freedom of movement was important to them. In some cases, as with Sally, removing breasts meant greater physical freedom and this was seen as valuable in setting standards for young women.

As supportive as many children were of their mothers and grandmothers, others found the postmastectomy period emotionally trying. Karen's youngest son had a particularly difficult time with her decision to live flat; he had been still nursing until shortly before her diagnosis.

> When we're snuggling, getting ready for bed, sometimes he'll say something like, "I really liked the milk I used to drink from your breasts" or something, and I'll say, "Oh, yeah, you know, I really enjoyed that." That was a good experience for us. . . . So he'll just say something small like that on occasion, or he'll say, "Remember when you were squishy?" You know, like, right after my surgery he was calling my chest "no-boobs." And he would be, like, "I don't like your no-boobs." I mean it hurt my feelings terribly. I mean he was—you know, he was just about to turn three when I had the mastectomies, and he's like, "I don't like your no-boobs," and, you know, "You need to get them back." And "You need to grow them back." And I was like, "No, I'm not going to grow them back, this is how they are going to be."

Even though Karen's son lamented the loss of her breasts, it was her older son's fears that she might die that produced the greater concern for her.

> My older son struggled a lot and continues to struggle a lot. My father-in-law died of prostate cancer about a month before I was diagnosed, and

> so he still says things like "Grandpa had cancer. Grandpa died of cancer. Mommy had cancer." And he's just, like, waiting. . . . And I'm like, "Not everybody who gets cancer dies from cancer," but he has anxiety about it. My husband travels a lot, and whenever he's gone my son just has massive anxiety. I talked to him about it, like "When Daddy would come and go [before the diagnosis] you were fine," and I ask him why he's upset. And he's just told me straight up, "Well, that was before you had cancer. What happens if Daddy is away and you get cancer?"

Karen's younger son's sadness was overshadowed by her older son's concerns that she could die. Like Karen, many women I interviewed understood mastectomy to be the best insurance against dying from cancer, thus allowing them to be fully present as parents.

The relationship between breast cancer and parenting involves a range of emotions. The women in this study feared death and were anxious about the impact a future cancer might have on their bodies and also their families. Breasts were often very significant to women as physical markers of motherhood and femininity, but being a present parent was far more important. Children sometimes helped to normalize a woman's new body while intimate partners struggled. Both BRCA-positive women and women with breast cancer believed a long life without the anxiety of cancer was worth the physical sacrifice in order to be fully present for their existing or future children. Breasts are deeply connected to mothering, but one can mother effectively without breasts.

Conclusion

The women who told me their stories arrived at the decision to undergo a prophylactic mastectomy through the complex relationship of personal identity, fears about health risks and death, and attention to the impact on those closest to them. Despite explaining their decisions as distinctly personal choices, participants often talked about the cultural expectations for women's bodies, their difficult interactions with health care providers as spokespeople for the institution of medicine, and their concern for how others would perceive their bodies. That is, the decisions women made were not designed to resist the gender structure or the power of medical authorities; nor were they designed to conform. Women made decisions that best suited their personal situation, but these individual decisions were always made in relation to the broader social context. In the interactions leading up to and following their mastectomy, the women were constantly shaping and being shaped by the cultural ideologies that permeate the entire gender structure. In the next chapter, the discussion of embodied resistance and conformity amplifies our understanding of how individuals navigate gender in their lives after breast cancer treatment.

We often take for granted that certain physical traits are essential to intelligibly gendered embodiment. Gender theorists suggest that unless we adhere to dominant norms of embodiment, we risk gender policing, various kinds of sanctions (including violence), and other issues. There is great pressure to be accountable to the norms; to act outside them is often theorized as an act of resistance or rebellion, of creating gender trouble. However, women indicated to me that their decisions to act outside of the norm were more about creating a livable life than about resistance. It was about imagining something new, and about having that new way of being be visible and accepted by those around them.

In explaining their decisions around prophylactic mastectomy, these women indicated that breasts are not only symbolic of femininity but are also physical representations of the social structures of gender. Within sociology, we think of structures as those features of collective life that organize all aspects of our interactions and identities but also provide constraints. In this chapter and the next, the ways women talk about their breasts reinforce the idea of breasts as a physical manifestation of the gender structure. The acceptance of prophylactic mastectomy as acceptable for women who are BRCA positive is a relatively recent development. Less than ten years ago at the time of this writing, Angelina Jolie faced public scrutiny by physicians for choosing a bilateral mastectomy after her BRCA diagnosis. As will become even more evident in the next chapter, ensuring that women have breasts is important to many in the medical community, regardless of whether it is important to women themselves.

Chapter 3

Returning to Normal

Recovering from breast cancer can be a fraught process for both women and men. Gender identity, one's sense of one's body, and concerns about how that body will be perceived by others impact how individuals make sense of their recovery. Within the culture of breast cancer in the United States, recovery is primarily about restoring femininity in particular ways. In this chapter, I explore the stories told by participants regarding their decisions about breast reconstruction and experiences of recovery that both support and resist narratives of recovering the feminine body as central to the healing process. Further, I investigate the ways in which ideologies of masculinity can intervene in the recovery process for cisgender men. These narratives reflect how decisions about the recovery process can both reproduce conventional ideologies of femininity and resist limited understandings of what it means to be a woman or man or to have a gendered body.

Of the thirty-three women I interviewed, fifteen chose to have reconstruction, and eighteen did not. Women who lived flat tended to reflect deeply on their decision both before and after having mastectomies whereas the majority of women who chose reconstruction explained that it was simply part of the process. Many of the women who chose reconstruction described this surgery as a normal step in the recovery process, unworthy of contemplation at the time of diagnosis. When I asked how they had decided to have breast reconstruction, many participants responded that no other alternative had occurred to them. Delving deeper with all of the women I interviewed revealed complex relationships among their identities, their bodies, their social networks, and their sense of accountability to cultural norms.

Although the recovery outcomes for participants differed, their stories held common elements that illustrate the ways that visibility and intelligibility contribute to the achievement of gendered biolegitimacy. This process entails building a sense of bodily integrity, understanding one's body as authentic to one's past and present identity and experiences, returning to normal activities (particularly sex), and adjusting to the way that one is perceived by acquaintances and strangers. In the first part of the chapter, I focus on the ways that participants make sense of their decisions about recovery through narratives of integrity, self-recognition, perceptions of strangers/acquaintances, and concerns for current or potential intimate partners.

Options for Reconstructive Surgery

After having a bilateral mastectomy, women face a series of decisions about breast reconstruction concerning the timing of reconstruction and the type of reconstruction. In some cases, timing is determined by the medical team of surgeons and oncologists in coordination with other aspects of treatment, including radiation and chemotherapy. There are also several types of reconstruction to consider. The most basic is to live flat. That is, after a mastectomy that removes all breast tissue, the incisions are closed and left to heal. Women can then choose to live flat, wear prosthetics (foam or rubber forms that fit inside specialized bras or clothing with pockets) or alternate between the two. Alternatively, women can undergo surgical procedures to construct the form of breasts. It is important to note that men who have had breast cancer expressed similar recovery stories to the women participants, but they lacked access to the range of reconstructive options offered to women, a point to which I return in the next chapter. Of the women who participated in this study, two out of the thirteen women with BRCA diagnoses lived flat, and eleven had or planned to have breast reconstruction. Of the twenty women who were diagnosed with breast cancer, sixteen chose to live flat, and four chose reconstruction.

One common method of breast reconstruction involves placing tissue expanders (silicone pouches) under the pectoral muscle at the time of mastectomy. After a period of general healing, women then return to the plastic surgeon on a regular basis (as often as twice a week) to inflate the expanders via saline injections of two to four ounces. This process helps stretch the skin in preparation for breast implants. At the end of a predetermined period (generally four to six months), saline or silicone implants replace the expanders (figures 3.1 and 3.2). This procedure may be accompanied by nipple reconstruction or the tattooing of a nipple. Another reconstruction method involves transplanting a patient's own tissue to create the form of a breast (i.e., reconstruction with

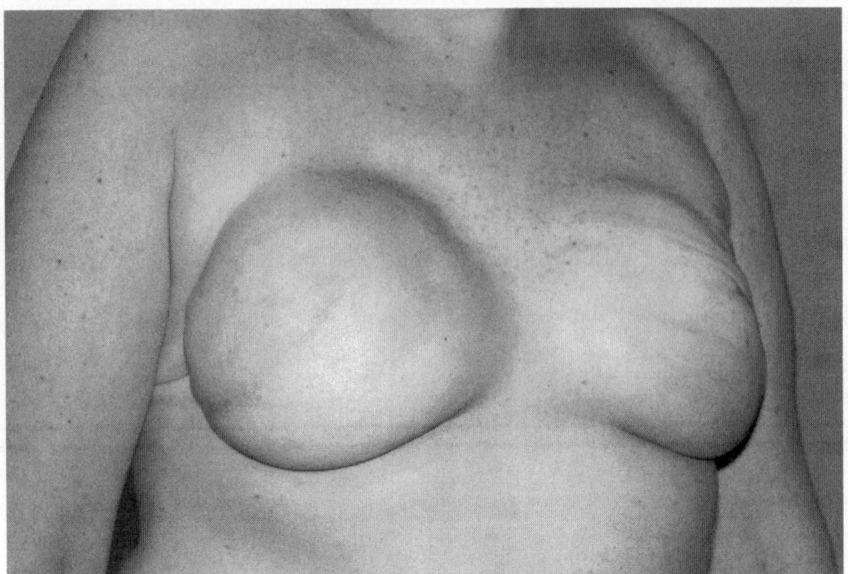

Figure 3.1. Breast reconstruction using silicone implants and expanders after bilateral mastectomy. Image courtesy of medicalimages.com

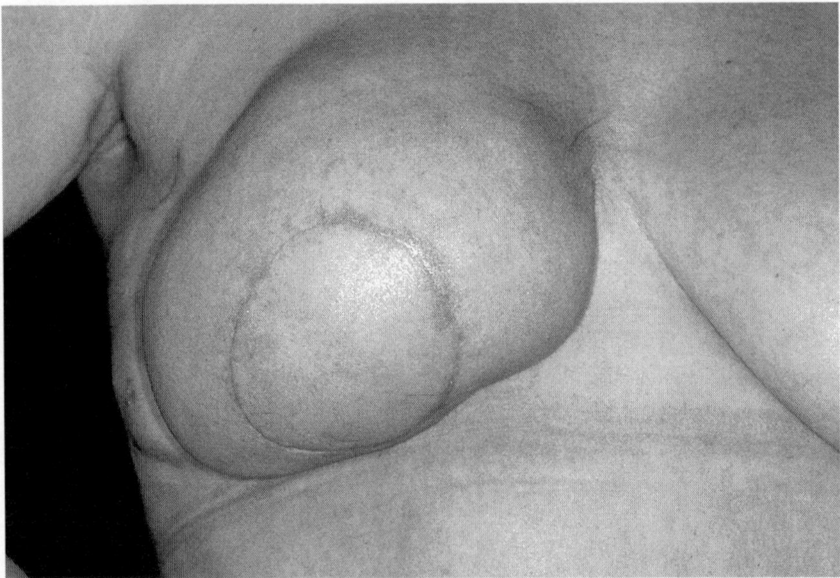

Figure 3.2. Breast reconstruction after single mastectomy using the deep inferior epigastric perforator (DIEP) flap procedure. This is repeated on the other breast in the case of a bilateral mastectomy. Image courtesy of sciencephoto.com

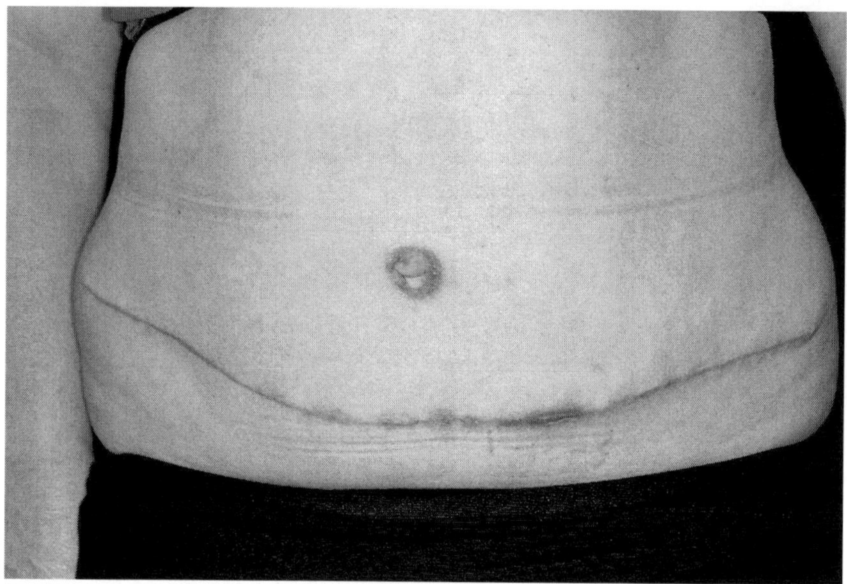

Figure 3.3. Abdominal scarring after a deep inferior epigastric perforator (DIEP) flap procedure. Image courtesy of sciencephoto.com

autologous tissue). In short, muscle, fat, and skin are "donated" from one part of the patient's body (typically the abdomen, buttocks, thighs, or back) and used to reconstruct breasts (figure 3.3). Implants can also be added to these procedures.[1] These are all intensive procedures; the overall complication rate ranges from 5.3 percent to 46.4 percent depending on various health factors, the cancer treatment plan, and the type of reconstruction chosen (see Brooke, Mesa, and Uluer 2012; Jagsi et al. 2014; Sullivan et al. 2008).

Women participants used similar language to describe their decisions, even though the outcomes were different. Regardless of their reconstructive choices and the range of factors influencing these choices, a sense of bodily integrity and authenticity were the backdrop against which reconstructive decisions were made. The term *integrity* commonly refers to the quality of being honest and to a state of wholeness; however, the stories told by cis women in this research use "integrity" to include a definition that is more fluid, plastic, and full of possibility. Understanding integrity in this way can even include the incorporation of "alien matter" into the human body (Shildrick 2010). *Authenticity* is closely connected to the concept of integrity. Whereas integrity refers to the physical state of the body and one's understanding of that body as whole, authenticity refers to a woman's sense that her body is genuine and true to her own character. More expansive self-definitions of bodily integrity and the generally broad definition of authenticity allow both women who live flat and those who choose breast reconstruction to draw on these themes as they construct their personal narratives of breast cancer within the context of cultural expectations about female bodies.

The most basic of these cultural expectations is the normality of a breasted body. A body with reconstructed breasts was seen by those who chose this option as nice, natural, or normal. That is to say, breasted bodies are authentically female. According to Colleen, a breasted body was symbolic of coming through BRCA or breast cancer "unscathed or sort of whole." Sam also equated "normal" with "whole." Her decision to have breast reconstruction was based on a desire to "feel normal again in some way, more whole physically." The repetition of terms like "whole" and "normal" belies the importance of the physical body to a sense of self. This is the crux of authenticity. Both flat and breasted women wanted to feel whole and normal after surgery. Having breasts after bilateral mastectomy was construed by participants who chose reconstruction as a return to an authentic—that is, "normal" female—body. Those who chose to live flat alternatively explained that due to the addition of synthetic materials to the body or the removal of tissue from other parts of the body to construct breasts, reconstruction was incompatible with their sense of authenticity.

Madison felt that breast reconstruction made it possible for her to recognize her body after bilateral mastectomy for BRCA: "I did always really like my body. I didn't want to be in a situation where I felt completely uncomfortable in my own body and didn't look a way that was recognizable to me." Although Madison had "no interest in cosmetic surgery," her perspective shifted after receiving her test results. The surgery helped her body seem authentic to her in a way that a flat body would not.

Cosmetic surgery has been at the crux of many feminist debates about gender and the body (see Davis 1995, 2003, 2009; Dull and West 1991; Heyes and Jones 2009; Morgan 1991; Negrin 2002). Choices about cosmetic surgery, including breast reconstruction, occur through a balance of a woman's sense of self and her relationship to gender expectations about women's bodies. Typically, women expressed gender expectations through the language of normalcy. Looking normal or "good" meant both recognizing oneself after bilateral mastectomy and being recognizable as a feminine person. As Margaret explained, feeling normal was also connected to her self-perception: "I just wanted to get back on my feet and as close to normal, based on how I looked and felt. I mean, they don't look the same [as before], but I guess I feel more comfortable in my own skin. . . . It represented some kind of normalcy to have something rebuilt there." Although Rachel observed that "you can never replace what you had naturally," she chose reconstruction because "it made me feel like I was still a whole person."

Underlying the concept of feeling whole is the reaction to disease. Wholeness signifies moving past the diseased state and returning to health. Margaret, who chose implants, told me, "I don't know if I'm ready to look at myself with that much of a reminder, you know with nothing there at all." Colleen expressed similar sentiments: "[Living flat] would be a really harsh daily reminder that this traumatic event had happened." For these women and many who chose to reconstruct breasts, seeing something on their chest besides a scar was about returning to a normal appearance after mastectomy. These women did not want to see "battle scars," as some describe the marks of mastectomy. Instead, they wanted to return their breasts to an idealized state and thus diminish their fears of the breast as a trigger of cancerous memory and future anxiety. These concerns never fully leave, but they may become less apparent for some women when there is not an obvious visual marker.

Integrity

In contrast to the authenticity drive that resulted in breast reconstruction, a rhetoric of integrity was often crucial to women choosing to live flat. Integrity encompasses both a sense of a body that is free of technological intervention and one with full muscle function. Linda, for example, held the view that reconstruction used "foreign bodies . . . [or] cannibaliz[ed] good parts to make things that kind of look like breasts." In Linda's view, both reconstructive options—expander and implants or autologous/ flap procedures—compromise a woman's bodily integrity by adding foreign material to the body or taking away from other parts of the body.

For many who live flat, sacrificing function for appearance was unacceptable. Karen was one of several women who were uncompromising in their desire to retain their normal muscle function.

> The whole process of putting something behind your pec muscle and slowly expanding it, painfully, to stick some other foreign object in your body or maybe take some other part of your body and put it in there, it all feels really strange. Especially because you don't get back sexual function or breastfeeding ability. So all of that is so that you can make other people comfortable with how you look. And I know that's not how it is for everyone, like for other people they need to be comfortable with how they look, too. But it turned out I am comfortable with how I look. It's other peoples' issue sometimes.

Karen's statement makes clear that there are two central factors, in her opinion, that figure into decisions about reconstruction: (1) a woman's comfort with her body image and (2) the body's function. How people feel about their body after reconstruction may include a consideration for how they are viewed by others. For Karen, this concern was less relevant than her postmastectomy physical capabilities.

Sandy was especially concerned about muscle function after bilateral mastectomy. She said, "I like my muscles the way they are. I am a competitive athlete. I am scrawny enough that the only reconstruction they could have done would've been the expanders, and do not mess with my pecs, thank you very much! Alternatively, if I had the body fat, I wouldn't have wanted my core disturbed for a TRAM. I would not have wanted someone to play with my lats. Breasts are so much less important to me than having the integrity of my muscles." The importance of muscle function was a concern for many women after breast reconstruction.

Following mastectomy, individuals experience a loss of sensation in their chest and an inability to breastfeed. Breast reconstruction also severely limits muscle function. TRAM flap procedures impede the function of the remaining chest muscles, the transplanted muscle tissue, and the muscles at the donor site. The use of expanders and implants also limits the function of pectoral muscles, though not as severely as transplants.

Like the women who live flat, Jody (who lives breasted) was wary of the TRAM flap procedure because she "didn't want to lose access to those muscles." In addition, she expressed some sadness that she was not fully informed about the loss of functionality from expanders: "I wish I had known that I was not going to have as much use of my pectoral muscles. It's more of an inconvenience than it is an actual hindrance." Several women described this inconvenience in terms of their inability to open jars or to slice hard objects such as carrots.[2] This physical hindrance did not lead Jody to regret reconstruction, but many women who live flat found the idea of compromising any muscle function to be simply unthinkable.

Along with a concern for physical functioning, women who live flat explained that having foreign materials or rearranging tissue is appalling and not worth the end result of conforming to normative standards of female bodies. Edie had a fierce reaction when her doctors offered up options for breast reconstruction: "I remember thinking, not on my fucking life! I mean the idea of having foreign material under my skin is a hideous thought to me. And then when I realized that for the surgery, they actually disconnect your pectoral muscle to stick the silicon under the muscle I was like, are they fucking kidding me? I mean, not only does it hurt like hell, but [women who do this] have diminished function." The combination of pain, the fear of losing muscle function, and Edie's visceral reaction to foreign material rendered breast reconstruction impossible for her. Sandy also felt that breast reconstruction was "too insulting to the body," given the added risk of infection and the pain associated with the procedure.

An insult to the body is, specifically, an affront to the body's integrity. This sentiment is evident in the frequency with which women who live flat expressed that their bodies had been put through enough. Kate, who initially had implants, "deconstructed" her breasts after a string of complications. She articulated the commonly held feeling among flat women that her body was threatened by medical procedures:

> You kind of feel like you want to own something and you need some agency, right? So it's like, all right, I'm losing the breast, I'll get back the breast. I'll do reconstruction. Like, people tell you, you know, you do chemo, you lose your hair, but it comes back. You're not prepared that you're metamorphosing, right? You're kind of thinking you've got to get back to where you were. You're hanging on to life here, and you think that life as you have known it before is better than the scary life that's being proposed. [After the complications with reconstruction] I was just like, enough. Enough. Stay away from my breasts. Or lack of breasts. Stay away from my body. I don't want anything invading—it was awful.

Kate posited reconstruction as a return to her physical state before mastectomy. Like regrowing hair after chemo, Kate believed that her health care providers presented breast reconstruction after mastectomy as a procedure that would restore her body to normal. Once the reality of reconstruction set in (the unnaturalness of the "mounds" and the health risks of complications), Kate had to rethink bodily integrity. She became adamant about reconstruction as threatening, feeling strongly that physicians needed to stay away from her breasts. At the same time, she was evolving. Her understanding of the connection between her identity and her body shifted to a place where reconstructed breasts were not in line with her sense of self. Further, Kate raised the issue of agency. In making decisions about reconstruction, women are confronting cultural ideologies and the ways in which those ideologies have been institutionalized through medical practice.

Kate was critical about the reality of reconstruction as a way to meet cultural ideals: "You're basically getting mounds put in so that your form looks the same to the outside world. But what's really there when you look naked in the mirror will no longer be anything that resembles the breasts that you've grown up with." As Kate's observation suggests, our decisions about our bodies are never purely the product of individual choice. These decisions are also a matter of presenting ourselves to the world at large. This does not mean that there is only one influence or one outcome. Rather, individuals make choices considering the various influences on, values of, and meanings about gendered embodiment as they relate to our own personal histories of gender.

Past experiences of bodily identification were important to Edie as she made sense of her decision to live flat after mastectomy: "The way I look now is how I looked when I was eleven. I mean, I remember looking like this. I remember feeling well while looking like this. I remember being happy while looking like this. To me, it's not that big a deal." Edie's harkening back to adolescence is important as the onset of puberty is a physiological marker of becoming a "real" woman. In his study of transgender men, Henry Rubin asserted that the physical changes (breast growth and menarche) that occur during puberty can be particularly distressing for trans men because these changes mark a transition via "the physical and hegemonic criterion for adult womanhood" (2003, 99). Before puberty, the bodies of boys and girls are visibly similar in most interactions. Edie's return to her adolescent understanding of her body is an act of what Kelly Underman has called "affective disposition, a particular way of feeling embedded in a cultural context" (2015, 180). To make sense of the physical changes wrought by bilateral mastectomy, women who live flat have to rethink their relationship to their cultural context. Before puberty, the women who live flat generally thought of themselves as female without question. This experience provided a model for reconciling their new, flat body, with their gender identity. Kate and Edie both described the end result of the process by which some women attempted to align their embodied identities with a cultural context imbued with normative expectations about women's bodies.

Like the women who live breasted, the act of recognizing one's body and being recognizable to others remained important to the women who live flat. In other words, the visual effect of reconstruction played an important role in deciding what physical form their body would take after bilateral mastectomy. Many women who live flat were somewhat critical of being overly concerned with appearance. Sadie, for example, asserted, "Reconstruction is not reconstructing anything. It's putting an unfeeling lump of something on your chest so your clothes look better." Similarly, Catherine felt that choosing breast reconstruction was linked to a desire to comply with societal norms about what a female body should be. For her, the complications of additional surgery were too great a risk simply for the purpose of regaining a normative form: "I would love to see the shape of breasts on my body, but no, I am unwilling to do what it takes to have that. I mean I did talk to them about different types of reconstruction, and I don't have enough body fat. I don't want to put my body through the multiple surgeries it might take to get it back, and I'm unwilling to move tissue from this place to that in order to, I don't know, conform. And I do feel that it is an issue of conformity."

Living flat opens space for a critical examination of standards of feminine beauty. Several of the women who live flat conflated conforming to gender norms with vanity, and they attempted to distinguish their personal interest in a visually appealing body after mastectomy. Many were careful to explain that they were not particularly interested in makeup or fashion. Their examples of vanity included stereotypically feminine behaviors—that is, they established that they had a history of physical nonconformity. Despite this, looking good was important to most of the women who live flat. Karen stated, "I think I look good. [Breast reconstruction] seems like a lot to go through just to look a certain way." Reconstruction was cast as a vain choice, yet living flat remained aesthetically pleasing. Many who chose reconstruction were proud of their appearance. Catherine, for example, did research on living flat and found self-portraits by a photographer who had done so. "She had taken some topless pictures of herself on a beach, playing with her children, and her results were absolutely beautiful. So I decided at that point to go bilaterally flat."

That women who live flat see their bodies as beautiful creates a stark contrast to how they view reconstructed breasts. Many women turned to the internet to research images of reconstructed breasts. Women like Edie were appalled by what they saw: "The first thing I did was to go look for reconstructed boobs on the internet . . . I started looking at these things, and I'm like, holy shit, because to my way of thinking this stuff looked horrific. I mean, we cancer ladies, we like to call them 'Frankenboobies.'" Ashley also commented on "the Frankenstein-ness of how they look when they're done." Similar sentiments were expressed in subtler ways. Rather than monstrous, Linda felt that reconstructed breasts simply do not live up to the expectation that they will look like natural breasts. "The thing is, these are not breasts. They do not make breasts. They make things that kind of look like them, but they are not breasts. They are dead lumps." These women emphasized that reconstructed breasts are just lumps of material, whether synthetic or transplanted from other parts of the body. As Kate researched reconstruction options after some complications with expanders, she decided that the aesthetic of a breasted body was not desirable: "I'm learning that it's just sticking mounds on my body. And then they tattoo nipples on. I'm like, why do I need that? If I need a tattoo, I'll get one on my ass."

These sentiments were tied to a fairly widespread disdain for vanity and a preferential focus on function. As Ellen explained, "What's the point? There's no feeling, they are ugly, you don't get your nipple. So what's the point of having boobs for vanity purposes?" Many who live flat balanced aesthetic considerations with issues of functionality. In other words, if reconstructed breasts do not function as natural breasts, and if they are unappealing visually (at least without clothes), then why bother? When I asked why she did not choose reconstruction, Fran responded simply, "Why have it?" For the participants who live flat, reconstructed breasts meant conforming to cultural norms. Reconstructed breasts also failed to live up to their aesthetic standards. The disdain for vanity and decision to live flat were connected to a strong undercurrent of independence. That is, these women insisted that they do not to look for approval from others regarding their decisions about their body, nor do they require others to affirm their bodies as beautiful. Edie explained that in deciding to live flat she did not consult her husband. She asked his opinion only after she had made up her mind: "I would never ask him [if he'd like me to have breast reconstruction]. I told him at one point after researching that I had more or less decided that I probably would never get reconstruction. I asked him if it bothered him in any way. And he said, 'Oh for God's sakes!' And then he said, 'Look, I would prefer you don't have reconstruction.' He's shit-scared of anesthesia; he doesn't like me put under. He also doesn't like silicone boobs. He associates it with transvestites [laughs]." Clearly, women like Edie care about how their intimate partner will react to their decisions to live flat, but this concern does not extend to changing their minds if the partner objects. Edie's decision began with her relationship to norms of feminine beauty and her assessment of her husband's reaction simply reinforced her decision rather than swaying it.

In addition to being centrally about how one is seen by others, vanity is also connected to beauty. For women who chose to live flat, reconstructed breasts cannot be beautiful, but flat chests can. Even though women who live flat embrace a narrative of independence and personal choice, it is rarely this simple in practice. The perceptions of others do matter to both those who live flat and those who reconstruct. It is also important to many women who live flat to effect change in public perceptions of postmastectomy bodies.[3]

The cultural pressure on women to pursue beauty is immense. Even as women who live flat insist that they make this choice in contradiction of beauty norms, personal aesthetics and the importance of beauty are still strong forces with which women contend.[4] Women who choose breast reconstruction and those who choose to live flat both rely on a narrative of aesthetics that contrasts with a narrative of vanity. The concepts of beauty and vanity are contested within feminist scholarship (see Bordo 1993, 2009; Davis 1995, 2003, 2009; Felski 2006; Furnham and Swami 2007; Gagné and McGaughey 2002; Gimlin 2002, 2007, 2010, 2013; Jain 2013; Stuart and Donaghue 2011). From these debates, there has been an evolution in feminist understandings of beauty from "the rhetoric of victimization and oppression to an alternative language of empowerment and resistance" (Felski 2006, 280). Beauty thus becomes a powerful discursive tool that can be deployed in the construction of self-identity, as was the case for the women in this study. Avoiding the language of vanity in favor of aesthetics is a way for women to set themselves apart from what many find to be the often problematic relationship between cultural beauty norms and the culture of breast cancer awareness (King 2006; Sulik 2011). Beauty remains important to the women who reconstruct their breasts and the women who live flat. The distinction, according to those who live flat, lies in whether one is primarily concerned with one's own body image or how that body appears to others.

Conversations with these women revealed that regardless of how participants use the language of normalcy and naturalness to explain their decisions, women who have mastectomies end up with modified bodies. According to Catherine, no matter what choice a woman makes, she chooses some type of reconstruction. "I chose a nonconventional reconstruction, and conventional being reconstruction. I didn't get the shape of breasts on my body, but if you think this isn't reconstruction, you're kind of crazy. I reconstructed my body. This is a form of reconstruction." Kathy felt quite similarly: "I've had a woman say recently that she got reconstruction immediately after getting her mastectomy and she said she was so happy she still had a chest. I still have a chest. Just because I didn't get reconstruction doesn't mean I don't still have a chest."[5] Both Catherine's and Kathy's statements reflect the sense that, at least temporarily, breast cancer alters one's sense of integrity, of completeness. When women make decisions about reconstruction, they primarily act in ways that help them regain a sense of an integrated body and which reflect their sense of themselves.

Still, these choices often come down to a woman's understanding of her embodied identity and her relationship to femininity. Samantha, who lives flat, came to this understanding by participating in a public art installation on self-image that involved having her naked torso painted. She described this as incredibly important to making sense of her body and identity after mastectomy: "I stood there for four hours while [the artist] painted me and answered people's questions. I was there to show people that regardless of what your body is going through, you can still be whole . . . I need to put myself out there and go, 'Okay, I'm still a woman.' I still can feel like a woman and in fact feel more feminine than I've ever felt. It comes from inside, not outside." For Samantha, the feeling of wholeness, of authenticity, was not specifically tied to her decision about reconstruction. Rather, it was intrinsically about her self-image and her understanding that this self-image is connected to her own perceptions, rather than those of others.

Emily, who lives breasted, was also reflexive about this process, saying, "It would be great to say that I'm strong enough as a person and have this identity completely separate from my physical self, but that's not the case." Although Samantha and Emily had different physical outcomes, they both described a process whereby women reconcile their choices about their bodies with feelings of femininity. Strength here can be understood as a process of becoming. Samantha expressed insecurity about living flat, but her participation in the art installation served as a catalyst for rethinking what her body meant for her identity as a feminine woman. Although mastectomies and reconstruction may be a threat to bodily integrity, how a woman incorporates these changes into her sense of self is a strong indicator of her choices about reconstruction.

Flat or breasted must both be thought of as forms of reconstruction that reflect a woman's sense of bodily authenticity. Traditional reconstruction requires additional emotional work because it necessitates including foreign substances into one's definition of bodily integrity. Both choices require that women grapple with feelings of authenticity and integrity in order to determine what level of intervention they can accommodate while retaining or reimagining an identity with which they are comfortable.

Self-Recognition

Women who live breasted also described their fears about recognizing themselves after surgery as well as having others view their bodies positively according to the idealized female body. This was a determining factor in Michelle's decision to have reconstruction after a prophylactic bilateral mastectomy: "I'm [young] and I am single, and I'm going to have these boobs the rest of my life. I need someone who's going to do a damn good job at making me look as good as I possibly can. . . . A lot [of my decision] was what I'm going to have to look at in the mirror every single day . . . I wanted to look good in clothes, of course, but also I wanted to not be totally freaked out looking at myself in the mirror." The naked aesthetic is not only a significant reminder of the trauma of surgery but also reflects the internalization of normative expectations about what a female body should look like. Choosing breast reconstruction in many ways indicated a degree of personal affinity and attachment to this norm.

Michelle's statement also indicates that it is not just the appearance of the naked body that matters for women. Jody acknowledged that her reconstructed breasts would look different from her biological breasts. For her, the clothed appearance was the greatest concern. "I just wanted to have something there. That's pretty much it. If not for my peace of mind, but for the ability to at least fit in some clothes . . . I don't know if I'd like to have nothing there, because I kind of have a belly. I need to have something there. At least for me . . . I never intended my reconstruction to go very far, just to have basic mounds." The phrasing of "basic mounds" suggests that Jody's concern is not with the naked form. Instead, the importance of a breasted shape is to improve the fit and appearance of clothes and to mask her belly, which she felt would be unpleasantly prominent without breasts. Rachel also emphasized the importance of clothed appearance over naked appearance: "I always felt that if I could just look decent in clothing and not have to wear a prosthesis that was going to be just fine for me . . . [as long as] nobody would know the difference [when I was clothed]. That was really all that I was concerned with." For Rachel, clothed appearance was important in deciding how to reconstruct her postmastectomy body. Although prosthetics would have provided the shape she desired, they would have limited the variety of clothing she could wear. These comments suggest that women who chose to reconstruct their breasts wanted to retain the typical feminine form while clothed and to have some semblance of the naked appearance to which they were accustomed.

For some women, feeling whole also meant making choices that honored the importance of breasts in their life before cancer. Rather than focus on the visual impact of having a breasted body, Nicole emphasized the affective importance of her breasts.

> It's not because I'm worried about how I'm gonna look afterwards or anything like that. It was solely because [my breasts] *mean* something to me, and it's because I've breastfed my children and I loved breastfeeding them. . . . It was, wow, the breasts that fed my children are no longer gonna be there when I have this surgery, and that's what gets me . . . I found out they've started doing surgery a little differently so they'll still kinda look the same. I'll feel like they're mine. [And] hopefully I can have the nipple sparing surgery, so at least I'll still have a part of me, the breasts that fed my children.

As a BRCA-positive woman, Nicole had the option of a nipple-sparing mastectomy. This is largely unavailable to women with breast cancer. Nicole believed that retaining her nipples would help her stay connected to her experience of breastfeeding, which was integral to her self-image. For Nicole, femininity was not simply a matter of aesthetics, but also incorporated the experience of motherhood. Adding silicone implants did not threaten her bodily integrity because keeping her nipples allowed her to integrate the foreign material into her sense of bodily authenticity. Further, nipple retention meant that, for Nicole, a critical component of her embodied history as a mother remained physically present.

The ability to incorporate foreign material into one's self-perception was distinct to the women who chose breast reconstruction. Madison reported that her tissue expanders "totally feel a part of" her, even though "they're really hard and they don't feel natural." She thus expressed a sense of authenticity (that the synthetic material of the expanders is part of her) while simultaneously acknowledging that her bodily integrity was compromised because the implants felt unnatural. Michelle was quite candid about the unnaturalness of tissue expanders. Instead of painful, she described them as fun: "It was kind of hilarious to like just be laying there and watch [the expanders] pump up and see your breasts get bigger right in front of your eyes. . . . It kind of became an exciting process just because with each step you're a little bit closer to being done." While Michelle specifically meant being done with the reconstruction process, her statement also indicates an end point in identity work, when her physical form would allow her to return to her old self. This process of reidentifying with one's body is a response to cancer's recidivism. It is a form of affective protection against the possibility of a recurrence. To have breast reconstruction after a prophylactic bilateral mastectomy is a return to normal feminine embodiment that belies the body's history of cancer.

Although they framed the issue of symmetry and aesthetic appeal in terms of self-image rather than social perception, these themes resonated with many women as they described their rationale for pursuing bilateral mastectomy. Fran, for example, expressed a desire to have a physical form that she found personally appealing after treatment. Like many women in this study, Fran's assessment of the aesthetics of her breasts before breast cancer impacted her decision to have a bilateral mastectomy: "One of [my breasts] I liked, and one of them I didn't like [laughs]. The one I didn't like had an inverted nipple and was kind of weird, and the one I did like is the one that had the diagnosis . . . it seemed ridiculous to me to just have one off and not the other. Especially since the other one I didn't like anyway. . . . Now that [breast cancer] screwed up my good boob and I have this bad boob left, so it was like, just get rid of it all."

Fran had a very clear sense of personal aesthetic value for her breasts. For her, a bilateral mastectomy was more aesthetically pleasing to her than the alternatives of lumpectomy or unilateral mastectomy. Similarly, Maggie found the idea of having one breast unacceptable. "I can't deal with asymmetry. I couldn't really picture myself having one big boob and one flat side. That was not reconcilable in my mind whatsoever." The ability to look at one's body after breast cancer treatment and see an image that was identifiable as herself and aesthetically pleasing was deeply important to many women. The personal visual appeal of their bodies and the connection between their body and their sense of self, apart from the perceptions of others, were major motivations to pursue bilateral mastectomies.

For many women, issues of symmetry were essential in deciding to have a bilateral mastectomy. Describing this feeling, Alison says, "I figured if I had a single mastectomy and didn't have reconstruction, to then just have one breast, you'd either always have to wear a prosthesis or go around being uneven . . . I felt that either way [with or without reconstruction], it would be easier to achieve symmetry by having a bilateral mastectomy." Alison's aesthetic concerns combined with her concern about future cancer risk: "I just didn't want to have to deal with it again in the future. I know this is contrary to what the research is telling us, that you know there isn't a greater risk of getting cancer in the other breast, but I'm thirty-two, that's plenty of time for something to sneak up on me." Other women made their decisions based on the ways in which physical symmetry aligned with aspects of their identities. Catherine stated, "As an artist, I can say without qualm that symmetry is important to me." As Linda stated, "symmetry is gigantic." For artists, athletes, and many other women, symmetry was a critical component of their decision to undergo mastectomy, yet it is a factor that the medical profession is il- equipped to manage.

Edie expressed great concern for the visual results of her surgery in terms of shape generally rather than symmetry specifically: "I come from a long line of artisans and artists and architects. I am not an artist myself, but I am very, very visual. How things look is important to me. And not from a vanity point of view . . . I don't wear makeup; I don't care that I have wrinkles, for example. But certain things, especially shapes are important." Her visual concerns about her postmastectomy body are strikingly different from the assumptions surgeons make about aesthetics. In her experience, "[The first surgeon] thought that the reason I wanted a double mastectomy was for reasons of vanity. So that I would get a better reconstruction. . . . You know when they tell you, 'You need a mastectomy,' they expect you to get all upset about that, from the feminine vanity point of view. So it's usually presented as . . . 'Don't worry we can fix you up right away.'" The language of symmetry, in contrast to that of vanity, was particularly important to those who chose to live flat, a point to which I will return in the next chapter. Vanity is tied to expectations about femininity and to an aesthetic for others, while symmetry is about a personal aesthetic. Vanity also relates to the understanding among medical providers that women choose mastectomy to achieve a better reconstructive outcome (see Gross 2015). Those women who wanted to live flat needed a different language for explaining that the visual effect of surgery mattered to them, but not in a way that reinforced norms of feminine beauty.

Several women with BRCA diagnoses pursued bilateral mastectomy for reasons that Edie characterized as vain. For women with BRCA diagnoses, a prophylactic mastectomy (often, but not always, conducted with immediate breast reconstruction) produced more desirable aesthetic results than a similar course of action after a presumably inevitable breast cancer diagnosis. Importantly, the women who had reconstruction did not use this better aesthetic outcome to justify having bilateral mastectomy. Rather, it was seen as a secondary benefit of having the surgery, particularly by young, BRCA-positive women. Megan explained, "You get to keep the nipples this way, and for the most part my breasts will eventually look like they always have." Nipple-sparing mastectomies are controversial because of the possibility of developing breast cancer in the nipple tissue, but they remain an option for young, BRCA-positive women. In contrast, after a breast cancer diagnosis, nipple-sparing mastectomies are not an option. Megan had a pleasant perspective of her breasts before her diagnosis, so retaining her nipples meant retaining the physical aesthetic to which she was accustomed.

The disjuncture between patient concerns for aesthetics and surgeon's assumptions about patient vanity create conflict when discussing bilateral mastectomies within medical care. The women in this study made a clear distinction between aesthetics and vanity when discussing their mastectomies. The women's view of vanity as negative derives from their understanding that vanity is connected to how one is perceived by others. Colleen made this point clear in discussing her bilateral mastectomy performed after her second breast cancer diagnosis. Her initial lumpectomy left her dissatisfied with her appearance. Colleen noted that the difference between her breasts "wasn't super noticeable, but it was noticeable to me and I always felt this subtle irritation at that difference." Colleen elaborated, stating, "With my clothes on probably no one else noticed . . . but I noticed and it bothered me." Colleen and Edie both emphasized the fact that they are not worried about how they appear to others; rather, they wanted to have bodies pleasing to their own eyes.

In her research on cosmetic surgery, Kathy Davis argued that women who undergo cosmetic surgery are not merely "cultural dopes" or "robots" acting in naive accordance with cultural norms (1995, 2003). That is, they are not simply trying to reshape their bodies to meet conventional standards of feminine beauty but are making decisions that help bolster their sense of self for themselves. In this study, women's resistance to vanity and their subsequent, individualized aesthetic framing of the visual outcomes of surgery support the view that the choice to have a mastectomy contradicts cultural norms about feminine beauty.

As Edie's statement shows, doctors are as susceptible as anyone else to these beauty norms. When she asked for a bilateral mastectomy, Edie's surgeons assumed she was anticipating reconstructive surgery and she wanted this surgery in order to yield more aesthetically pleasing breast reconstruction. In fact, many of the women in this study chose bilateral mastectomies with an express desire to live flat. Regardless of a woman's desire to live flat or have breast reconstruction, women repeatedly expressed that symmetry was central to their ability to build a positive body image after surgery.

Accountability

The relationships between social accountability and being visible to others were explicit across many narratives. Kate, for example, believed that decisions about reconstruction are about "having your body presented to the world." For Margaret, the presentation of her postmastectomy body in daily life was central to her decision to have breast reconstruction.

> I think about how okay I would be with not having any breasts and just having just a flat chest. And I would probably, you know, I would be okay with that, but I feel like it would make other people uncomfortable. If I'm being honest, I feel like I'm kind of sacrificing what I would choose if I was just choosing for me alone. I feel like I am making a choice based on other peoples' comfort level more than I am my own.

Similarly, Karen worried about making "someone else feel uncomfortable" as a result of her decision to live flat. She went on to explain, "I don't want to be the woman that makes people not know how to look at her." At the same time, she wondered whether she *should* push the comfort zones of strangers in order to provide greater visibility for women who live flat. At stake in this concern for making others uncomfortable is a sort of accountability crisis resulting from living flat. By living flat, women choose to reject the ideals of embodied femininity to which they are culturally accountable (West and Zimmerman 1987, 2009). Karen acknowledged that this alternative embodiment may make it difficult for strangers to determine her gender, thus making them uncomfortable (Westbrook and Schilt 2014).

Additionally, there is a sense of accountability not to gender norms but to other women who live flat. In this way, Karen suggests that by presenting her flat body to others, she may contribute to increasing gendered biolegitimacy for others who live flat by increasing the visibility of this type of embodiment. Such visibility is critical given that visible physical characteristics remain the initial criteria used in most face-to-face interactions (Friedman 2013; Kessler and McKenna [1978] 1985). Shifting how bodies are perceived can impact the ability of others to be recognized. Although transgender and gender nonconforming individuals may experience the tensions inherent in gender accountability on a regular basis, living flat can shift heterosexual cisgender women from a place of taken-for-granted accountability to a place of ambiguity.

Kate described an instance during which she was uncertain about how her body was being read: "I wore a white T-shirt one day [to the gym]. I mean, you could really see my form. I don't have breasts, so it's not like it's anything I thought anybody would be paying attention to . . . I'm on the stair stepper, and I look out and this kid is videotaping. I was like, I don't know why this kid is videotaping me. Like, is it just funny because I'm a middle-aged lady exercising? Is it funny because I look completely bizarre to him?" Kate never confirmed the rationale behind the videotaping incident. Her suspicion that her body was the catalyst for the teenager's interest is a testament to the ways in which visible gender accountability matters not only in interactions but simply in public spaces. Kate did not interact with the teenager; he was simply a passerby who caught sight of her. By entering a public space, individuals are subject to gender assessment. For women who live flat, this can create situations that they do not know how to navigate because they expect and want to be viewed by others as women. Living flat can make this more difficult and even result in "interactional breakdown" (Schilt 2010; West and Zimmerman 1987).

Some women found that their concerns about visibility were unfounded. Linda initially wore prosthetics to spare the sensibilities of those around her. This was often uncomfortable for her, and she would invariably take off the prosthetics by mid-day. Linda explained, "Many days even when I was wearing them, I'd get halfway through the day and I couldn't stand it one second more, and I would run to the ladies' room and rip them off. So I came to work wearing breasts, and I'd go home flat. . . . Nobody died. Nobody fainted. Nobody died. Nobody had a heart attack. They all survived, it's okay." Breasts are construed as critical visible markers of femininity, but Linda's experience showed her that her chest was less consequential for her professional experiences than she initially expected. For Emily, by contrast, losing this marker would constitute the loss of her identity: "I mean it sounds simplistic, but I think that it really is—it really does come down to the fact that society defines a woman as a human who has breasts. And I think it's kind of like subconscious wiring of, well, I am a woman, and a woman must have breasts, so if I don't have breasts, I'm not a woman. So I think it would've felt like I was giving up that aspect of my identity if I didn't have reconstruction."

Several women who chose to live flat reported that they could separate their personal sense of femininity from broader normative ideals. Karen explained, "I want to be a woman who doesn't need breasts to still feel sexy or desirable or to feel feminine." After a great deal of reflection, she decided that she could, in fact, be the woman she wanted to be and chose to live flat. Samantha was quite clear that even though society expects women to have breasts, alternatives exist: "I'm still a woman. I still can feel like a woman. In fact, I feel more feminine than I've ever felt, and it comes from inside, not outside." For those women who found that they felt as feminine, or even more feminine, than before surgery, there was a process of first acknowledging the cultural imperative to have breasts, followed by releasing oneself from that expectation. When asked if she faced any resistance to her choice to live flat, Maggie said, "Most of the resistance I got was from other breast cancer patients. Like, 'Why did you decide to do it that way? How can you do that? How can you like your body that way? Like, seriously?' And then, also, the other side to that is a lot of women are jealous. They're like 'God, I wish I could be comfortable without boobs.' And I'm like, 'Well, that's interesting. Why don't you just be comfortable without boobs?'"

For many women, the pressure to have breasts is too great to consider any alternative. Participants reported that this pressure manifested through interactions with doctors, through constant images in the media, from family, and from acquaintances. Seeing oneself as somewhat at odds with mainstream culture was a significant consideration in the decision of some women to live flat. Catherine articulated this point in terms of a feminist consciousness. "It's feminist for me. It's the right decision for me, but that's not to say that you cannot also make the feminist decision to reconstruct your body. But it's the questioning, I think, that would apply to the word feminist, the ability to question." A feminist consciousness or any perspective that promotes questioning the status quo can release some women from the physical expectations of femininity. A feminist perspective is not necessarily predictive of a woman's choices regarding mastectomy; rather, it is the ability to question taken-for-granted assumptions about feminine bodies that allows some women to live flat.

The decisions women make about reconstruction occur within a cultural context where, in every interaction, individuals are expected to remain accountable to gender norms so that others may determine their gender with ease. In addition, cultural expectations presume that women will have two breasts and that these breasts are necessary to support a feminine identity. Choosing breast reconstruction allows women to remain accountable to these expectations while living flat challenges the norm. Importantly, living flat did not always create interactional breakdown, nor did it prevent women from cultivating a feminine identity. Regardless of their choice, women often assessed the social impact of their decisions against cultural expectations of what women's bodies should be.

Scars

Women who live breasted are supported in this process by constant improvements in surgical technique. These advancements were particularly significant for those women who had seen family members go through breast reconstruction after bilateral mastectomy. Emily had watched her mother go through breast cancer treatment before her own BRCA diagnosis. When her mother had a mastectomy, the cosmetic options were far less advanced.

> Whereas [my mother] had a scar straight across her chest, the surgical option that I had, you really can't even tell. Once the scars heal you can't tell that you ever even had a surgery.[6] So that was a game changer for me, that cosmetically I would still be pretty much normal.

For Emily, a highly visible scar was a symbol of illness and a non-normal body. Scars mar the visual integrity of the body, and for many women they create an unappealing aesthetic. Appearing not normal may reinforce the initial feelings of cancer anxiety that led to a bilateral mastectomy.

Reducing the visibility of scars through improved surgical methods is critical for women like Colleen.

> I think the technology piece did play a role . . . I did spend some time, reading about the technology, asking a lot of questions about the aesthetic piece because that was important to me. It definitely made the decision easier when the plastic surgeon said, "Your body's really going to look the same, you're going to just have small scars kind of under your arms. . . . It's not going to be a huge scar across your chest." Once she said that, it sort of clicked for me.

For Colleen, it was both the visibility of scars and her concern that reconstructed breasts would look significantly different than her biological breasts that caused aesthetic angst.

Aesthetics thus incorporate multiple concerns for those who reconstruct breasts, such as whether the reconstructed breasts will look normal. Madison was particularly concerned about whether her breasts would look normal: "I was like, 'Oh my God, I'm going to be disfigured. And I'm not going to look like a normal woman, and I'm going to, you know, look like a weird crazy person under my clothes, and everything's going to suck forever.'" Breast reconstruction was Madison's insurance against appearing like a "weird crazy person" when naked. To not have normative breasts under one's clothes is here considered antithetical to being a normal woman.

Although most of the men in this study discussed their mastectomy in matter-of-fact terms, several described the emotional difficulty connected to their surgically altered bodies, referring to their bodies as "alien." Experiencing one's body as alien complicates the notion that mastectomy is a simple decision for men. Ed tried to explain what it felt like to lose sensation in a part of his body.

> The appearance felt alien for a bit. I'm looking at something that's not part of my body, and initially I didn't want to touch it because of the sensation there. You know, when I did touch it, it wasn't me because I couldn't feel anything. But clearly it was me, so there was a little divorce from that—a little separation from that side of my body for about a month. It just happens to be there on me but isn't really me. But now it's me, you know. I'm pretty comfortable with it being there . . . I'm feeling around to make sure I can feel other parts, and then as I touch into that area I know I'm touching it, but I don't feel it on my chest. I can feel my finger touching something, but I don't feel the responsiveness. I don't feel my chest. . . . The first word that came to mind is dead part of the body or unresponsive part of the body. . . . It's a part of me, but a part where there's no sensation.

The lack of sensation is a common issue for male and female breast cancer patients. Even though many men don't identify with their nipples, losing physical sensation in any part of the body can be an unsettling experience.

Along with a lack of feeling, mastectomies often result in significant scar tissue. This is the case for both men and women after mastectomy, but there are significant differences in the embodied experiences of healing. Often men were able to ignore their scars because chest hair covered them. Regardless of chest hair, men typically are not offered any reconstruction options whereas women are strongly encouraged to undergo this additional surgery.

Larry believed that the nonchalance concerning mastectomy was the product of how men are supposed to feel about their bodies, rather than reflective of the actual experience of breast cancer. He also connected reconstruction with cultural associations between women and breasts that render invisible any connection a man may feel to this part of his body:

> The comment was made to me by a variety of people that, well, I guess it's not such a big deal to have breast cancer for men because you know, they don't identify as women do with their breasts and all that, and it's true, you don't—first of all you don't deal with the reconstructive issues, decision and issues. Because generally in men, you know, you don't do reconstruction. I still get out of the shower every morning and you know; my body is altered. So, there is still a psychological aspect of you know, having the mastectomy.

Ed described his chest as concave after mastectomy, yet no physician offered an implant to fill the space. Most men in the study had difficulty imagining why a man might want reconstruction. Ed mentioned reconstruction to his surgeon as a joke. He followed this story by stating, "If it were important to my career, if I were a trainer as I see in the gym, I'd want [reconstruction], I want to look good for prospective clients, current clients." Only Tim discussed considering any kind of reconstruction.

> When I was first diagnosed and everything, I did meet with a plastic surgeon . . . to talk to him about it, and he was like, "Well I've never really done anything for a male, but you know, I can tell you the options of this," this and that, and everything, you know, the reconstruction of it. They take skin and they try to, like, grow a new nipple, or you'll get it tattooed back on or whatever. After I met with him and stuff, you know, I kind of let that sink in. I was, like, that's just a lot of weird, whatever, you know what? After surgery and stuff, this is going to be my battle wound. This is a battle that I fought. I won. I really don't want to forget about it, so that's what it is.

Tim was the youngest man interviewed and had a job where his chest would be visible to others. He and Ed both expressed concerns that some men might be professionally impacted by a disfigured chest. The shift from viewing his body as disfigured to viewing it as imbued with battle scars signifies a masculinized perspective on breast cancer.

Even though the men in this study eschewed a macho identity, the language of battle scars allowed some of them to interpret their scars not as markers of breast cancer but as markers of survival. A narrative of survivorship and battle scars is present in breast cancer culture at large (Mukherjee 2010; Sulik 2011). For men, it is a distinctly masculine way to connect with that culture.

Accepting and reinterpreting scars was important for male breast cancer survivors because reconstruction generally is not an option for men. Frank's surgeon told him, "'You're a man. We'll remove the breast, and that will just be the end of it.' For a woman, he said there'll be other issues, but they are usually not an issue for a man. That would be the end of the discussion." Larry's surgeon told him that reconstruction "is available but generally men don't do it." His surgeon described one patient who was a swimmer and chose to get a nipple tattoo. This was the most common option for men, but no men in this study chose to get one. Most found the idea of a tattoo humorous. In describing his scar, Ezra said: "It's a very nice scar. It's as unobtrusive as a scar like that can be. . . . I'm still contemplating getting some kind of nipple tattoo, but I'm not sure yet. I'm kidding [laughs]. Only if I can put something rude there [laughs]." Ezra went on to say that a tattoo was just "too much" and wondered, "Who would see it anyway?" Men in this study found little value in tattooing. Other forms of reconstruction were vaguely understood by men and offered little in terms of their personal comfort with their chests.

Men also expressed concerns about how others would react upon seeing a scarred chest. Across interviews, it was clear that appearance matters to men, but the imperatives of masculinity create a context that encourages them to reconcile their concerns quickly. Ed was concerned about how his clothes would fit after surgery and was relieved that his small stature helped mask the concavity present after mastectomy: "I'm a small guy . . . in the past I always thought that was a disadvantage. Turns out to be an advantage. I can wear any kind of shirt I want whereas a bunch of the men I see at the gym I go to, if they wore my clothes, they'd look awfully funny if they had a mastectomy." Ed was worried about how he looked because he did not want to "cause people any queasiness." Frank expressed concern that "people would look at [him] funny," so he wore a shirt while swimming for two years after surgery to prevent causing strangers unease. Rather than focus on others, Frank described his feelings of shame about his postsurgery body. "I'm deformed . . . I'm a man that's missing a breast. I'm a man that had breast cancer. . . . And I'm deformed." Over time, his feelings of shame gave way to a sense of acceptance. Where once Frank feared people staring at him, he eventually took pride in his appearance: "I want them to look at me, and I want them to come up and say, 'What the heck is that?' So I can make them aware that there is such a thing [as male breast cancer]."

Other men denied that physical appearance mattered much to them. For Larry, it "was not a body image thing." Ezra similarly stated, "I'm way past the age where physical appearance is a big deal." For both Larry and Ezra, deemphasizing body image was connected to their advancing age. Larry talked about how young, "pumped up" men might be more focused than are older men on the appearance of their chests. Yet each of these men described various feelings of discomfort after surgery. Owen compared the body image issues of women and men with breast cancer: "I don't think it's as big an issue as it might be. I don't think our issues are that much different from the women except for the whole issue of reconstruction which we don't really have to worry about. There is a certain amount of body image, you know when they cut you up, you're cut up. And for men it—or at least for me—it took a year or two before I could go on a beach without a T-shirt and be comfortable enough to wander around."

Concern about appearance after mastectomy for men focused primarily on scarring. Owen had a particularly disfiguring surgery. Upon examining the incision, his primary care physician exclaimed, "Jesus! They cut you in half, didn't they?" It is difficult to imagine a male physician saying this to a female patient. Normative ideals of masculinity create a sense of presumed distance between a man's identity and his body. While mastectomy scars are initially jarring, men like Owen felt that the mastectomy scar "is what it is," and it does not require a great deal of attention. Men reported intimate partners, both male and female, being uniformly supportive, assuring them that they "look great" after surgery.

Mastectomy is a defining experience of breast cancer for most men and many women. The surgery is framed by breast cancer activist culture as particularly detrimental to normative femininity. Men therefore do not have a ready narrative via breast cancer culture to help make sense of their experience. Instead, they can rely on masculine tropes that encourage them to not get caught up in their body image. This is not to say that masculinity is protective against body image issues; rather, hegemonic masculinity places pressure on men to "both achieve culturally privileged bodies at the same time that they are interpellated to maintain a functional, aloof, and distanced relation to their bodies" (Norman 2011, 432). The body is thus a resource by which to access or lay claim to the privileges of hegemonic masculinity. However, the emergence of "aesthetic masculinity" prioritizes bodies that appear young, strong, and vibrant (Atkinson 2008).

Given that the average age of men with breast cancer is sixty-eight, some of the pressures of aesthetic masculinity are lessened (American Cancer Society 2018). As Henry pointed out, "I'm getting to be middle aged. I don't spend a lot of time admiring myself in the mirror." In addition, the scope of what counts as an acceptable male body is fairly broad, with everything from scars to "dad bods" (i.e., a slightly out-of-shape figure) portrayed in the popular media as acceptable. For the men in this study, so long as they did not discomfit others, their postmastectomy bodies could become unremarkable over time. Making sense of their scars in this way is also protective for men, given that reconstructive options are incredibly limited for them. Being able to distance themselves from aesthetic concerns is a mechanism for managing the relative lack of medical options for constructing a chest that resembled what they had before breast cancer.

The idea that scars make other people uncomfortable was very important to women as well as to men. In the previous chapter, I referenced Catherine's desire to make scars and flat chests beautiful as well as Judy's husband's inability to view her scars. Unlike men, women's chests are typically not publicly visible. Scars, for women, tend to be more of a personal concern rather than a fear about making strangers uncomfortable. Gender norms require women to keep their chests covered, so while both women and men are concerned about scars, the public nature of this concern tends to differ.

The acceptability of publicly visible mastectomy scars became national news in 2012 when Jodi Jaecks petitioned the Seattle Parks and Recreation department to permit her to swim topless in public pools after her double mastectomy (Abbey 2012; Associated Press/Huffington Post 2012; Reilly 2012; Valdes 2012; Vaughan 2012). After her mastectomy, Jaecks took up swimming to stay healthy but was frustrated by the lack of bathing suits that would comfortably fit after bilateral mastectomy. Scars can be sensitive and painful to touch, and the seams in bathing suits can rub uncomfortably. Mastectomy bathing suits include prosthetics that can be cumbersome, uncomfortable, and inappropriate for someone who has chosen to live flat. Jaecks pursued her petition after being told that she could not swim at a public pool without gender-appropriate swimwear.

Swimming and bathing suits were brought up by woman and men as examples of moments when postmastectomy bodies created unease either for themselves or for others. Additionally, finding suitable swimwear was of particular concern for women. Only two women, Kate and Ellen, thought about swimming topless like Jaecks. After a long discussion about her frustrations about bathing suits that do not fit, and dog ears falling out of the side of bathing suits, Kate considered swimming topless but ultimately decided against it.

> In the age of YouTube and everything, I really am not trying to embarrass my [kids]. You know, my kids are ten and thirteen now . . . I have not done that [swim topless], but I'm very interested in it [laughs]. If it was just me and I didn't have to be concerned about anything that would be emotionally traumatic for my daughters, I would have already have been doing that all along. The idea of somebody taping me on a phone and then having, you know, a billion hits on something would haunt my daughters for the rest of their lives.

Ellen, in contrast, described the colorful, floral tattoo that she was planning to cover her scars as a way to have more comfort swimming topless in public spaces. She explained that without the tattoo she will swim topless in private spaces, such as a friend's backyard pool. The tattoo, for Ellen, was a way to cover up the scar, which was her primary concern.

> I'm afraid of offending people. I will say to people if we're at the house or if we're at someone's pool, "Does anyone care if I take my top off?" I want to ask first out of courtesy. I don't want to offend anyone. You know? They are scars. They are not pretty, but my chest actually looks really nice . . . I shouldn't hide. I'm proud of it. I'm proud of my scars. I'm proud of what I've been through.

For both Kate and Ellen, their primary concern in publicly showing their scars had to do with the sensibilities of others. Several men had similar concerns. Alan avoided swimming without a shirt for two years because he "didn't want people to look at me funny" and because "I was embarrassed and maybe a little ashamed that I had to go around with only one boob . . . I'm deformed. People will look at me. I'm a man that's missing a breast. I'm a man that had breast cancer. And just worrying about what other people are going to think."

Fear about how they would be perceived and shame were key factors in the ways that men and women experienced swimming. Like Kate, Ezra focused on the emotions of his kids. While preparing for their first beach vacation after his mastectomy, Ezra asked his kids, "'What do you guys think? Do you think I should just do what I usually do [swim without a shirt] or would you like me to wear a shirt when I'm on the beach?' And my son said he would prefer me to have a swim shirt on." Ed also wore a shirt while swimming; he stated, "I'm not uncomfortable with it at all," but he "wouldn't want anybody who might feel queasy about it see it [the scar]. I don't show it off." Although he spoke generally about other people's potential inability to cope with seeing scars, it was really his wife that he was concerned about because she "could faint over the sight of blood." When his wife and daughter bought him a surfer shirt, he wore it happily not only because it spared his wife's discomfort but because it protected him from the sun.

Men's scarred chests can become unremarkable in the sense that we, in the United States, expect men to appear topless in public, especially while swimming. While visible scars might make people uncomfortable, the relative infrequency and lack of awareness of breast cancer in men makes it unlikely that a stranger would assume that a man with a chest scar had breast cancer. Frank's statement about being deformed is directly connected to his sense that being a man and having breast cancer are incongruent. Unless the general public perceives chest scars on men as the result of breast cancer, it is unlikely that the discomfort Frank fears causing others will be realized. Alan and Tim each described using people's curiosity about their scars at the beach or swimming pools as an opportunity to educate strangers about male breast cancer. For women, though, publicly visible scars meant confronting norms that state that women should not be topless in public. Suzy rejected swimming topless explicitly for this reason. She said, "Flatness doesn't need to be normalized by being naked. I don't mind to a certain extent staying within the confines of expected clothing norms for women."

In an article for ESPN on Jaeck's story, Rick Reilly took issue with the initial stance of the Parks and Recreation department as well as with anyone who would be upset by a woman swimming topless after mastectomy. He wrote, "Is it too hard on our kids, on us, to see scars where breasts used to be? Are we that void of compassion that we can't stand to look?" (Reilly 2019). Mastectomy scars have very different meanings for women and men based on differing norms of appropriate embodiment and public comportment. When women who live flat appear topless in public, they are directly confronting expectations of women's bodies in public places. Stories like that of Jaecks and the concerns participants expressed about swimming topless in public are not about rebellion or resistance but about imagining how to live with gendered embodiments that do not fit normative expectations and about asking others to imagine along with them what other embodiments can be deemed legitimate. Scars become an invitation to others to perceive gendered bodies in new ways, thus creating new possibilities for gendered biolegitimacy because allowing scarred bodies (particularly women's bodies) to become visible provides a degree of legitimacy by rejecting the notion that such bodies are deformed, disfigured, or out of order.

Sexuality and Intimate Partner Concerns

In many cases, participants' concerns about how their bodies would be perceived centered on their identity as heterosexual women. Because gender identity, physical characteristics, and sexuality are interrelated (see Schilt and Westbrook 2009; Schwartz 2007), some women find their heterosexuality suddenly questionable. Whether women reconstruct breasts or live flat, the sexual pleasure that many once associated with their breasts disappears. After a mastectomy, the breast region loses sensation. Further, the reality of losing one's breasts causes some women, like Julie, to disconnect from their breasts.

> Breasts are a huge part of my self-confidence in terms of the way I look. They're a huge part of my sexuality. They've been a focal point of the way I have presented myself sexually to the world [pause]. I don't really

> consider myself to be very sexual any more. I consider myself to be pretty asexual at this point. I don't want them touched. I don't want them looked at. I don't want to think about them. I don't know how it's gonna turn out, and I'm quite worried about it, and I wonder if I'm ever going to feel sexy ever again [pause]. Part of me feels resigned to the idea that I would ever be sexually attractive [crying] ever again, or that I would never be. It's just something I have to accept. I'm quite worried because it's like I don't know how freaked out men are gonna be to be with a woman who has reconstructed breasts. I have a partner of seventeen years, and he never mentions any sort of disgust at the idea, but at the same time I don't know what he's thinking and it worries me.

Here, Julie's breasts are conflated with her identity not only as a woman but also as a sexy, heterosexual woman. For heterosexual women, sexual attractiveness to men is a defining component of both the gender category "woman" and heterosexuality (Schwartz 2007). Reconstruction was not an obvious solution to Julie's problem, as she was uncertain that reconstructed breasts would promote a return to (hetero)sexual attractiveness. Although reconstruction often involves some of the same techniques as breast implants for women without breast cancer, the visual results may be different. Most notable is the lack of a nipple on the reconstructed breasts of BRCA-positive women or those who have had breast cancer. Not only are breasts implicated in a woman's sense of heterosexuality, but there is also a particular breast aesthetic that is acceptable. Without nipples, reconstructed breasts do not live up to the ideal.

Julie was in a long-term relationship at the time of our interview. Other BRCA-positive women like Michelle who were single were especially concerned about how breast reconstruction would impact sexual relations. She worried, "I'm so young, and the guys that I'm dating are young, and this is not a normal thing, so I didn't know how a guy that I was dating for the first time would react or if it would be—if it would freak somebody out. I don't think that reconstructed breasts are terribly common at any age, especially at such a young age." Although Michelle expressed serious reservations about the reactions of intimate partners to reconstructed breasts, the alternative of living flat was unfathomable. Dating after reconstruction was conceivable to her, whereas dating while flat was not.

None of the heterosexual women in this study told me that their male partners wanted them to undergo reconstruction. These participants all expressed that their male partners' chief concern was their partner's well-being and that the decision was ultimately their own. Yet the women I interviewed often still couched their decisions about reconstruction through their interpretation of the expectations of male partners. Underlying their comments is the connection between heterosexuality, heteronormativity, and gender. In line with Sally's observation about the straight women in her social network, women in this study who chose reconstruction explained that they were concerned about the reactions of their partner and what he might not be saying. Amy, who was dating her husband when she was diagnosed with breast cancer, was certain that her husband "would never insist that I have reconstruction and I know that he loves me." Despite this certainty, she also stated, "I don't feel ready to do that [not have reconstruction] to him . . . I think it'd be hard on him. Sexually, I think it would be hard on him." Sociologist Pepper Schwartz argues that heterosexuality requires that individuals "are supposed to have certain kinds of bodies that reveal our heterosexuality" (2007, 84). Breast cancer and the decision to live flat have bodily implications that disrupt this supposition of a heteronormative social system.

In the previous chapter, I discussed Catherine's decision to spend as much time naked as possible so that both she and her husband could come to see her flat-chested body as beautiful and (hetero)sexy. By reimagining her body as sexy (i.e., desirable to her husband), Catherine was able to reinforce her femininity by virtue of its visibility.

> I almost feel even sort of freer without breasts and even more feminine, whatever that means. For me it almost feels like my body is even more feminine than I have ever been able to experience with breasts . . . I love being a woman. I love being female. I have always wanted to be flat-chested. Prior to meeting my husband, I dated women . . . I think that the gay, lesbian, bisexual community are just more open and willing to accept difference. Perhaps my ease in making this decision [to live flat], my comfort in making this decision, was influenced by my experience in relationships with women.

Catherine's past sexual history with women allowed her to see beyond the taken-for-grantedness of heterosexuality and prevented her flat chest from disrupting her sexual relationship with her husband. Catherine's practice of nakedness contradicted the sense of desexualization that Ellen felt. Pepper Schwartz (2007) links being desexed to being invisible, while Kristen Schilt and Laurel Westbrook (2009) note the role of visibility in de/legitimating the identity claims of trans people. The connection of visibility to sexual intelligibility relies on the relationship between the physical body and gender identity. Bodies, gender, sexuality, and visibility are intricately linked in the relationships discussed here. In this study, those women who had a bisexual, lesbian, or queer history reported that the physical changes to their breasts and the reality of living flat easier to manage than did the straight women.

Sally, who is married to a woman, was particularly interested in the role that sexual identity plays in making decisions about reconstruction. She told me that many women in her social network "talk about being a disappointment to their husband." She wondered if being a lesbian made it somehow easier to live flat. Sally's question suggests that there is a deep connection between doing gender and doing heterosexuality. Kristen Schilt and Laurel Westbrook argue "that doing gender in a way that does not reflect biological sex can be perceived as a threat to heterosexuality" (2009, 442). As such, those women who do not have to do heterosexuality in their intimate relationships may have greater flexibility in how they do gender, thus making the decision to live flat less problematic. For participants in this study, heterosexual relationships required a degree of emotional embodied labor different from queer relationships, through which women supported the masculinity of their partners and mitigated any potential disruptions to the heterosexual relationship that breastless embodiment would cause.[7]

Maggie, who is also married to a woman, identified as gender nonconforming. This identity generally made living flat easier for her: "Nobody could really tell my gender right off the bat until I opened my mouth. And so that I didn't mind at all. It was actually kind of nice to not have this assumption of, you know, a woman moving through the world." Maggie's gender identity did not automatically improve the sexual implications of her surgery and decision to live flat. Even though her breasts were not significant to her gender identity, the responsiveness of her nipples was important for her sexual identity. Maggie was unequivocal about her sexual attachment to her nipples. "My nipples were fabulous from a sexual perspective." Maggie's comments help to illustrate a critical contrast between heterosexual women and queer women. Ellen, Julie, and Michelle (all straight) embedded their sexual identity concerns in language about how their actual and potential male partners would react to their bodies. Maggie, although mentioning her female partner, was introspective and focused on her own feelings of being damaged, given that she lost a physical sensation important to her sexual identity.

Although sexuality is always relational, female heterosexuality is defined in terms of the male gaze and a woman's ability to be seen as desirable. Visibility is crucial to social life because "if [a woman] is not desired, she does not exist" (Schwartz 2007, 89). Visibility is not just about individual women, however. Rather, "looking and being looked at are fundamental steps in the process of establishing, perpetuating, or challenging social order" (Gagné and McGauhey 2002, 816). Women who are not bound by the norms of heterosexuality and binary gender are able to imagine new ways to remain visible and to bolster their gender and sexual identities. This reimagining of visibility and identity in turn constitutes a challenge to the social order. While both straight and queer women expressed reservations about how their partners would react to their bodies, these concerns were enough to cause some straight women to have reconstruction.

No matter what choice women make, however, the sexual function and appearance of breasts are compromised. Some women who choose reconstruction do so not because they want the form of breasts, but because they do not want to put their partners through any more difficulty. In other words, having reconstructed breasts is a way to keep intimate relations as normal as possible. These assertions are embedded in a structure of heteronormativity. Women who live flat accept that this supposed normalcy will never be achieved, and they work through it slowly with their partners. Kate likened living flat to the changes wrought on a body after childbearing: "I feel like I lucked out in feeling like a healthy, sexual, active human being whether or not I have breasts. [My relationship with my husband] is not really based on just the physical and breasts . . . I mean if we're in an essentially happy relationship and you have a baby and stretch marks occur, stretch marks are not going to be that big a deal on the other side of it. But if you're already in a relationship that's not so great anyway, then the stretch marks suddenly become somebody's focus."

Concerns about intimacy with one's partner reflect both the normative gender expectation that women have breasts and the normative expectations of heterosexuality that persons with "opposite bodies" will be attracted to one another. While lacking breasts in everyday interactions may go unnoticed, modifications to the breast become apparent in intimate encounters and disrupt both gender and sexuality norms. Regardless of the reconstructive choice women in this study made, most considered the impact of their decision on their partners—specifically, the sexual consequences. Reconstructive decisions were also deeply personal and rooted in how a woman understood the form and function of her body outside of sexual relationships.

Sexuality is relevant not only to cisgender women's decisions about breast reconstruction. Cisgender men with breast cancer also expressed sexuality-based concerns. Due to the associated complications for sexual virility, chemotherapy and hormone therapy (used in the treatment of estrogen-positive tumors) sometimes posed a threat to the masculine identities of the cis men in this study.[8] Several mentioned but were reticent to discuss in great detail the effects of tamoxifen on their libido and their relationships with significant others.[9] Ed stated simply, "It's been fine except for one thing [and] that is a decrease of libido [pause]. [My wife and I] worked through that, and we're fine." Ed declined to elaborate because he was at work and initially agreed to discuss the matter over e-mail, but he later decided not to comment further. Ted was concerned about this and other side effects of tamoxifen, and he was relieved when no side effects occurred. In our conversation he brought up a study he had read that states that 20 percent of men stop hormone therapy due to side effects, including weight gain and sexual dysfunction (Pemmaraju et al. 2012). Larry was among the most candid in discussing sexual dysfunction: "The tamoxifen, it definitely impacts your sexual desires and performance. Some men go off of it because of that. Some men don't ever go on it because there have been no clinical trials."

The combination of sexual side effects and uncertainty about its efficacy in men led many to avoid hormone treatment. Larry went on to say that tamoxifen impacted his sexual performance: "It definitely has an impact. I mean I'm sixty-seven, so you don't know whether [laughs], you know, a change is because you're getting older or what. But it is a real issue that I've had to deal with since the cancer diagnosis and the follow-up medication." As breast cancer typically is diagnosed in older men, their sexuality can be doubly impacted. Given the importance of sexual performance to masculinity, hormone therapy for breast cancer is one of the most problematic aspects of breast cancer care for some men. Virility is an increasingly important characteristic of the healthy male biocitizen (Gurevich et al. 2004; Loe 2004, 2006; Wienke 2000, 2005, 2006). According to the men I interviewed, the threat to virility caused by hormone therapy was one of the most difficult aspects of having breast cancer.

Both Larry and Owen discussed hot flashes as an unpleasant side effect of tamoxifen. Owen generally described tamoxifen treatment to be "a unique experience for men" due to the menopause-like symptoms caused by the drug. The side effects Owen experienced were compounded by his prostate cancer diagnosis four years after starting estrogen therapy for breast cancer: "The prostate cancer of course leaves you [pause], well, you're infertile, you're sterile. Not that I plan on fathering children, but psychologically it's just an adjustment . . . I think one of the hardest effects of prostate cancer [is] probably an accumulation of thirty years of diabetes, chemo and tamoxifen, and then prostate surgery, sort of the trifecta of erectile dysfunction." There was not much Owen's urologist felt would help the situation given his overlapping medical issues. According to Owen, "You're not able to have what people would consider a normal sex life. . . . It is what it is. You do what you can. You still have a lot of closeness. You have a lot of physical touch . . . you do what you can." Larry also emphasized alternative forms of intimacy. "With an understanding partner, cuddling can go a long way."

Sexual performance is an important component of masculine identity (Loe 2006). The side effects of breast cancer treatment on men's ability to have penetrative sex with a partner are perhaps the clearest area in which masculinity is threatened by breast cancer. This is evident in the inability of many men to discuss this aspect of their experience. Sexual performance also underlies some of the comments men with breast cancer heard from others. Henry's ability to father children was implicated in a question from an acquaintance: "I had one person who seriously asked me if my kids were my kids because he thought if I got breast cancer, I must have been some kind of hermaphrodite."

The implications of breast cancer for a man's sexual identity and the difficulty some men have in talking about this aspect of their experience are indicative of normative masculine identity. Sexual bravado is a socially accepted masculine behavior, but talking about one's inability to perform sexually (except in the context of commercials for drugs like Viagra) is a heteromasculine taboo. Admitting to sexual dysfunction, particularly if not combating it through the use of pharmaceuticals, is admitting to diminished masculinity. Although several men claimed that breast cancer did not threaten their masculinity, their statements about the sexual side effects of treatment suggested otherwise. The stories men told indicated a personal redefinition of the meaning and value associated with masculinity. Their narratives suggested that the ability to procreate and the ability to perform certain sexual acts are central to what it means to be a man and to the value of men's bodies. Yet as cis men redefine sexual intimacy (i.e., touch and cuddling instead of penetration) and disconnect fertility from masculinity, they present a challenge to the standard structure of gender.[10]

Conclusion

The narratives of participants in this research reaffirmed the centrality of gender to breast cancer recovery. However, these women and men show that normative expectations are not always the main drivers of patients' desires concerning their bodies after breast cancer. Decisions about breast cancer recovery emerge from concerns about one's health, body, identity, and social context. It is important to note that no woman in the study remarked that her choice about reconstruction was right for everyone. Universally, women who shared their experiences with me stressed that the method of reconstruction—whether living flat, living with prosthetics, having implants, or using one's own tissue to create breasts—is an individual choice based on how a woman reconciles the changes in her body with her identity.

The gender structure and femininity in particular powerfully influence the experience of breast cancer. Patients and providers must work within the institutional norms of the medical profession and in the context of the gender structure. At the same time, the very meanings of gender are being performed into existence through the experience of breast cancer, a disease that threatens commonsense ideas about femininity and its situatedness in the body.

When women choose to live flat, they fundamentally question the authority of the medical profession to singlehandedly determine the gendered biolegitimacy of female bodies, and through their position as biocitizens they assert their power to imagine embodiments that, to some women, feel even more feminine than they did before mastectomy. Additionally, the way that gender organizes relationships with others and/or constrains action was experienced by women in this chapter through their breasts. That is, the experience of having breasts and removing them is a physical manifestation of the ways that ideas about gender shape daily life. The prioritizing of certain aspects of these ideologies of gender is at the heart of tensions between patients and providers and is a critical component of the trouble that gender can cause for medical professionals.

Narratives about the interactions between postmastectomy patients and physicians highlight the important role ideas about feminine bodies play in defining physical and emotional well-being. Femininity was important to many women in this study, regardless of their reconstructive choice, but the narrow association of this trait with particular physical characteristics was shown to be faulty. Nevertheless, the commonly accepted association between visible physical traits and gender identity remains deeply influential in medical practice and was impactful for participants. The women who spoke about feeling more feminine while living flat explained their sensibility in terms of the visibility of their bodies. Women like Samantha felt liberated to wear more revealing clothing than they did before the mastectomy. Catherine described wanting to make scars sexy and desiring clothing that revealed a bit of scar. Although these women wanted to disassociate femininity from breasts, femininity remains a matter of the visible body. As these women reconsider how to do gender in everyday life, the visibility of their gender remains critical to their identities and daily lives.

Chapter 4

Ideologies of Gender in Surgical Cancer Care

In 2016, National Public Radio (NPR) and *The Atlantic* brought public attention to medical research suggesting that the patients of women doctors have lower mortality rates than patients of men doctors (Hamblin 2016; Schumann and Schumann 2016; Tsugawa et al. 2017). The media and social media attention to these findings took the predictable path of highlighting assumed differences between men and women. In the same issue of *JAMA Internal Medicine,* an editorial on this research suggested that the improved health outcomes documented by women physicians hinge on communication style, length of time spent with patients, and encouraging patients (Parks and Redberg 2017). Each of these characteristics is tied to stereotypical ideas about what it means to be a woman in society. This study and the brief flurry of attention it received are an opening into the complexities of the relationship between gender and medical care. The complexity stems from the various ways in which medical and lay communities define satisfactory health outcomes and the ways in which normative expectations about gender identity and embodiment are taken for granted yet are key determinants in medical decision-making.

Within medical care, the narrative around breast and gynecological cancers turns on stereotypes of femininity and female sexuality. Breast cancer care and activism specifically assume that there is a "right patient" for care: she is a cisgender, female-identified, heterosexual woman, with normative desires for her body's appearance. When a patient does not meet these assumptions, they create gender trouble for health care providers. As a result, the care of these cancers provides a unique window into processes of gender and embodiment within medical care (see, for example, Casper and Carpenter 2008; Hesse-Biber 2014; Oliffe 2009; Sulik 2011).

In this chapter I focus on the interactions between patients and providers with respect to three elective surgeries in cancer care: hysterectomy, prophylactic and contralateral mastectomy, and breast reconstruction. These elective surgeries illustrate how patients and providers rely on frames of health and gender to determine whether a given surgery is an appropriate option for cancer prevention or care. I use these cases of elective surgeries in gynecological and breast cancer care to explain how medical interactions are shaped by and thus reproduce ideologies of gender through the bodies of patients.

I understand these surgeries as examples of the tension between technologies of the self and technologies of power (Foucault 1988). According to Michel Foucault, technologies of power "determine the conduct of individuals and submit them to certain ends of domination" whereas technologies of the self "permit individuals to effect by their own means or with the help of others a certain number of operations on their own bodies, and souls, thoughts, conduct, and way of being, so as to transform themselves in order to attain a certain state of happiness" (1988, 18). As a technology of power, these surgeries serve to reinforce normative gendered biolegitimacy. As technologies of the self, these surgeries are interventions desired by patients in order to imagine new possibilities for gendered biolegitimacy and to craft their bodies into shapes that allow for the realization of livable lives.

In previous chapters I explored the ways that participants make sense of their medical decisions and their bodies with respect to their personal sensibilities, their connections to family and friends, and the perceptions of acquaintances and strangers. These are all key elements in achieving gendered biolegitimacy. The final element of importance in gender biolegitimacy is that of access to technologies of the body that create opportunities to alter the physical body in ways that do not necessarily conform to normative ideologies of gender. The differential access to these technologies and the rationale for permitting or restricting access is determined more by ideologies of gender than by the identities of the patients and providers in a given interaction. While clinical practice and medical decisions are supposedly determined through the principles of evidence-based medicine and patient-centered care, I show that ideas about gender can supersede both medical evidence and patient desires for their bodies during the care of gynecological and breast cancers.

Among the trans men participants, five men had undergone hysterectomies (one before transitioning medically and socially), and three were considering the surgery. All the trans men who participated in the study were aware that hysterectomy was a medically approved option even when they did not consider it a personal option. The participants ranged in age from twenty-two to seventy-one years old. The trans men and cisgender women who were BRCA positive tended to be younger ($n = 20$ under the age of forty). The majority of cisgender women diagnosed with breast cancer refused breast reconstruction ($n = 14$). The majority of cisgender women diagnosed as BRCA positive chose breast reconstruction ($n = 10$). Two of these participants had breast "deconstruction"; that is, they initially had breast reconstruction but later reversed the surgery to "live flat," which is the term adopted by cisgender women who forego or reverse breast reconstruction to have a flat chest rather than a chest with breasts. Four women in this study chose to have breast reconstruction after choosing a bilateral mastectomy.

Decisions about elective surgery in the case of gynecological and breast cancer highlight the tension between the foundational principles of clinical practice and the responsibilities inherent in biocitizenship. In the context of gynecological and breast cancers, ideologies of gender become central in resolving this tension. Patients who behave as biocitizens—by becoming informed about their options, the potential outcomes of a given procedure, and the risks involved in that procedure, and considering the impact on their quality of life—face obstacles to implementing their choices when these choices conflict with the ideologies of gender that serve as the foundation for medical understandings of evidence-based medicine and patient-centered care.

At various points in the cycles of "female" cancer care, doctors or patients may consider elective surgery. Each surgery involves the removal of currently healthy organs for the purpose of cancer prevention or the addition of foreign or transplanted material for the purpose of cancer recovery. These surgeries are differentially supported by the medical community based on whether the surgical outcome conforms to normative gender expectations. For medical professionals, the "decision to incision" must include clinical data and consider a patient's wishes. However, the stories related by research participants indicate that neither evidence-based medicine nor patient-centered care have been deciding factors for whether a health care provider promoted or rejected elective surgery. By comparing the decision to incision for these three elective surgeries, I show how ideas about gender can either help or hinder a patient's ability to access surgery depending on whether the surgery aligns a patient's body, identity, and normative gender expectations.

Principles of Medical Care

Contemporary medical care hinges on two key principals: evidence-based medicine and patient-centered care. These principals emerged in the 1960s and have become increasingly important, with distinct shifts occurring in the 1990s with respect to clinical research (see Armstrong 2007; Bardes 2012; Claridge and Fabian 2005; Sur and Dahm 2011). Until the 1990s, biomedical research was conducted primarily with white, male research subjects. Activists in the women's health movement and feminist scholars questioned this research model and pointed out how research standards led to gender-based disparities in health care access and outcomes (for a detailed history, see Ruzek 1978; Morgen 2002). As a result, clinical researchers have adopted an inclusion model in which women (as well as racial and ethnic minorities) are considered crucial to the research process (Epstein 2007; Mazure and Jones 2015). Practicing evidence-based medicine then means relying on data that were collected using binary and normative understandings of gender.

As the inclusion model became central to medical research in the 1990s, cultural competence and patient-centered care became linked in clinical interactions. Both the American Medical Association and the Institute of Medicine issued statements regarding "cultural competency," in which these groups argued that physicians and health care providers needed to understand the cultural assumptions that both they and their patients brought to medical interactions. Generally, the medical community understands cultural competence as a means by which to provide patient-centered care because the intention is to understand the cultural norms and values that inform a patient's experiences and interests with respect to medical care (Epner and Baile 2012; Saha, Beach, and Cooper 2008). Cultural competence is specifically used by the medical community in reference to disadvantaged patient populations and shares an emphasis on including patients in the health care decisions with patient-centered care (Bardes 2012).

Providing patient-centered/culturally competent care is implicitly linked to normative ideologies of gender, given that the medical community believes that providing patient-centered care requires being attentive to cultural norms (see Annandale and Hammarström 2010; Armstrong 2007; Bardes 2012; Claridge and Fabian 2005). The connection of both evidence-based medicine and patient-centered care to the women's health movement includes the implicit centrality of assumptions about gender in both components of medical care.

This is most evident in the approach of gender-specific medicine; the notion that every clinical decision, every diagnosis, every treatment must take the gender of the patient into account (Legato 2004). Gender-specific medicine reinforces a stark distinction between male and female bodies that cannot be crossed, and it defines appropriate medical care through these purported distinctions. Gender operates as a taken-for-granted system of not only physical difference but also culture that can shape the type of care patients need. Culture, in the medical community, is assumed to be part of a cohesive, fixed, identity shared by others occupying certain structural positions, including gender. Further, such a concept assumes that this position is an agreed upon, knowable, and immediately recognizable identity. In order to be patient-centered, physicians ought to know the culture of the patient and assume that their assessment matches that of the patient. In short, care cannot be patient-centered unless it also incorporates the gender ideologies of the culture around the patient. Similarly, care cannot be evidence-based unless the clinical research providing the evidence includes participants of the same gender as the patient.

Evidence-based medicine and patient-centered care are critical to the provision of medical care today. In the case of the three elective surgeries presented in this chapter, however, these principles fail. This failure is due to the ubiquity of gender ideologies in medicine and the implicit role of medical professionals to rely on and uphold gender as biopower. In other words, the medical community turns to gender norms as a means by which to assert control over the lives of patients when the medical evidence is lacking and the patients' desires resist the taken-for-granted norms of gendered embodiment.

Hysterectomy

In 2011, the American College of Obstetricians and Gynecologists (ACOG) released official statements in accordance with standards of care from transgender health advocacy organizations indicating that patients should have physical examinations for the body parts they have, regardless of the gender with which these parts are associated. ACOG's recommendation also acknowledged that lack of knowledge about trans patients may make providers uncomfortable administering these exams (ACOG 2011). What these statements neglect to acknowledge is the ongoing centrality of gender dysmorphia (colloquially, the experience of being "trapped" in the wrong body) to medical interactions generally and to gynecological care of transgender men specifically.

Originating in the standards of care promoted in the 1950s by physicians like Harry Benjamin, who were at the forefront of transgender medicine, the "wrong body" narrative serves as a gatekeeping tool for medical professionals treating transgender patients. These standards emerged from debates about the proper treatment of transgender people: is the goal of medical treatment to change behavior or change the body? Although the prevailing medical narrative advocated for changing the body, physicians willing to treat transgender patients would only consider those individuals who fit binary understandings of gender, largely to avoid malpractice suits and to fit transgender people into existing norms of gender (Meyerowitz 2002).

Central to the wrong body narrative is a "sense of profound alienation" between mind and body (Sullivan 2008, 106). Medical services are thus predicated on notions of right and wrong bodies as defined by normative expectations of embodiment based on a binary understanding of the gender identity of the patient, regardless of how individuals want to embody their identity. Given the widespread acceptance of this narrative, some transgender individuals use it as a discursive tool to gain access to medical services even if they do not personally identify with it (Bettcher 2014; Prosser 1998).

Several scholars have been deeply critical of this narrative and the way that it erases any embodied identity that counters a strictly binary view of gender (see Bettcher 2014; Johnson 2015; Spade 2003). The interpretation of the wrong body narrative as central to medical care for trans people implicitly reinforces the biopower of gender by marking some bodies as treatable and thus legitimate. Importantly, this legitimacy is enacted by medical professionals who work to align the gender presentation of their patients with not only visible secondary sex characteristics but also internal organs.[1]

ACOG's stance sets up a double bind for both patients and providers. Trans men are at once expected to reject the body parts associated with being female (that is, trans men are not expected to want breasts or reproductive organs that would allow them to bear children) but at the same time submit to medical care for those very parts. [2] Gynecologists, in turn, are implicitly trained to treat women as more than just a set of body parts. This sets up a double bind for both patients and providers. Trans men are expected (and encouraged through public health campaigns in some cities) to participate in Pap tests and pelvic exams yet are also expected to be uncomfortable with gynecological care due to a presumed sense of body dysmorphia. According to some physicians, the resolution to this double bind is to advocate for hysterectomy as an appropriate alternative to regular exams (Eyler 2007). Some physicians also recommend hysterectomy as an alternative to anxiety medication. Although surgery can be part of a strategy to avoid future medical risks (particularly cancer), removing organs is also a response to dissociation or disidentification as well as a permanent form of dissociation. Importantly, trans men in this study explained that while their personal concerns about cancer might motivate an interest in hysterectomy, physicians routinely offered the surgery even when transgender men did not initiate interest in it.

When trans men present for gynecological care, be it routine or emergency, their bodies can become untreatable. Regardless of whether a transgender man identifies with the wrong body narrative, this is the dominant paradigm through which medical professionals understand these men. Seeking gynecological care puts transgender men in conflict with a narrative that assumes they are uncomfortable with their reproductive organs and/or disidentify with them to the point of avoiding care. This is compounded by the fact that these organs and their care tend to cause others to identify an individual as a woman, thus unraveling the often complex biographical work transgender men have engaged in over time.

The clinical interaction between a health care provider and a transgender man may prove disruptive because the patient's identity and body and the provider's expectations and clinical space (defined by the expected woman-identified patient) do not align, thus making it potentially difficult for a provider to conduct the exam. From the medical perspective, the Papanicolaou test (Pap test) is an essential component of cancer prevention, so trans men must submit to this exam in the pursuit of health. The standards of care for trans men, however, recognize that pelvic exams may be "intolerable," and they link this intolerability to the low uptake of Pap tests among trans men.

Some practitioners interested in gynecological care for trans men tend to assume that these patients avoid the exam because it produces extreme anxiety and threatens their gender identity (Coleman et al. 2012; Eyler 2007; van Trotsenberg 2009). Although some trans men in this study did describe discomfort or dissociation during gynecological exams, all but one acquiesced to gynecological exams. The anxiety described by the participants was rooted less in how these trans men saw themselves or about the practicalities of the exam itself, and more in how they anticipated they would be seen or treated by providers. These concerns about treatment in medical settings reflect broader trends among transgender Americans. Discrimination against transgender patients within the medical community is well documented (Cruz 2014; Grant et al. 2011; Institute of Medicine 2011). Importantly, for many transgender people it is not the actual medical procedures that are concerning but the perceptions of and resulting treatment by medical professionals. These perceptions were described to me as critical sources of anxiety and concern with gynecological care.

It is useful here to remember Joe's concerns (quoted in chapter 1) that providers would perceive him as female because of his genitalia, despite all external physical indicators of his maleness (Joe was noticeably balding and sported a full beard). Isaac (also quoted in chapter 1) worried that health care providers' sense of shock upon seeing his body would impair their ability to treat him. So the concerns of trans men focused on neither the genitalia nor the actual examination procedures but rather on the providers' perception and how that would influence treatment. Although some research has suggested that trans men may experience physical discomfort or body dysphoria during exams, the distress expressed to me instead focused on the unpleasantness of the interaction during the exam and the need to mentally check out in order to cope with their understanding of how they were perceived by physicians.

Several trans men participants reported high degrees of anxiety when anticipating gynecological exams. Some took antianxiety medication to manage their emotional response to the exam. Joe explained that Ativan allowed him to "retreat into [his] own mind," and he described his experience of the exam in the following way: "I remember specifically saying, 'I'm checking out. See you guys later.' Letting the Ativan take over and just kind of not being present for it. [The doctor] did a great job explaining to me what she was going to do, but she didn't expect me to talk or interact. She seemed to know that I was gonna wall off in my own little protective fort in my mind and just try to disassociate as much as possible. That might not sound like so much that she allowed me to do that, but that was huge."

Although dissociation was described to me as a useful coping strategy by some trans men, some practitioners see this as something physicians should work to prevent. In an article written to provide clinical guidance to practitioners treating patients with histories of sexual trauma, Dr. Pamela Dole wrote, "It is important to help [the patient] in remaining relaxed and preventing disassociation" ([1999] 2001). The assumption that dissociation is problematic has roots, in part, in the changes to gynecological exams promoted by the women's health movement. However, the assumption within the medical community that dissociation is problematic for exams is highly normative and dismissive of the reality of these exams for some trans men. For the trans men who shared their stories with me, dissociation is about the health care interaction, not about their bodies, because it is the potential of these interactions to delegitimize their gender identity that they find distressing. In daily life, these trans men explained to me, they are comfortable with their bodies. Their identities, bodies, and the ways they are perceived by others are aligned, even if this alignment is different than normative expectations of gendered embodiment.

Again, it is not personal discomfort with their bodies (i.e., gender dysmorphia) but rather a discomfort with how trans men would be perceived by providers that has led to anxiety in the context of gynecological exams. The wrong body narrative obscures the possibility that discomfort in exams is about how trans men are perceived by health care providers, rather than personal discomfort with their bodies. Gabe described "having to be out of body" during medical treatment prior to a hysterectomy. This was not due to a deep body dysphoria but to his understanding of how medical professionals perceived him. He spoke at length about the harms that can occur during the experience of a hysterectomy. Gabe routinely saw his personal experiences repeated in his work as a hospital chaplain, where he had been in the position of advocating for trans men who are categorized as women upon admission to the hospital for hysterectomies. This meant wearing ID bracelets that categorized them as women, being placed in shared recovery rooms with women, and being verbally misgendered by hospital staff. These kinds of experiences suggest that patient identities and bodies are not always brought into immediate alignment by this particular surgery, even if providers assume that trans men desire hysterectomies.

Five men in this study had hysterectomies. Three men had hysterectomies before their medical and social transition, and two had the surgery after. Additionally, three men were seriously considering the surgery. Kevin explained that a hysterectomy was the answer to his concerns about insurance coverage for gynecological care and the actual exam itself.

> It's always a challenge, too, to know what to do with insurance and health care, and changing my gender marker or not changing it, and what does that mean for health care? And if my gender marker gets changed, are they going to be even less friendly towards me if I need any kind of care? Which is also influencing my own thoughts and decision-making around whether I want to get a hysterectomy. Because it's, like, if I keep these things, which I don't plan to do anything with them, not only will I have to keep going to see somebody every year or whatever, there's also a possibility that something could happen cancer-wise. And then, like, hell, forget that. I'll be seeing people all the time, and they'll be looking at stuff that I'm really not okay with.

Hysterectomy can be a welcome option for trans men who consider submitting to gynecological care to be a fraught experience. Even a trans man who is comfortable with gynecological care may consider a hysterectomy an easy "solution" to the assumed problem of gynecological care. Isaac regularly received preventive gynecological care throughout his adult life, and he was fortunate enough to find providers who were comfortable with both his identity and his body. As mentioned in chapter 1, gynecological care was important to Isaac because of his family history of endometriosis and gynecological cancers. Even though he was comfortable with gynecological care, Isaac eventually agreed to a hysterectomy after his gynecologist assured him that the surgery would be "an easy sell" to his insurance company because he was listed with the company as a transgender male and because of his family's history.

Joe and Isaac both had family histories of gynecological issues, including cancer. For Joe, a hysterectomy was a potential solution to both his fear of cancer and his concerns with pelvic exams. Joe was willing to endure a final pelvic exam because it would open the possibility for a hysterectomy that would ensure "not getting uterine cancer or having that risk any further and never having to undergo another physical exam again." Like Joe, Isaac had no actual physical complaints, yet his family history combined with his identity as transgender made hysterectomy a viable option for his physician because of the ease with which it would be approved by Isaac's insurance company not because Isaac had any indicators of cancer. For both Joe, who was a medical professional himself, and Isaac, health care providers strongly supported their hysterectomy as a reasonable option, despite the lack of physical indicators presenting an empirical rationale for surgery.

Chris was in a slightly different situation. He presented to his primary care physician with abdominal pain. During repeated visits over several months, Chris's physician brushed aside his concerns. After he was told several times that nothing was wrong, Chris was eventually referred to a gynecologist who told him, "'The good news is, you're not making it up.' . . . And then [she] asked me if I was later in life thinking about getting a hysterectomy at any point and recommended [a hysterectomy] because she had no idea what was going on." Chris's gynecologist recommended a hysterectomy because he was in obvious pain but she could not figure out the exact cause.

To prevent gynecological cancers, nine men in this study reported that physicians had recommended the removal of internal reproductive organs or questioned their interest in keeping these organs, despite the fact that trans men are not at increased risk of cervical cancer. It is important to note that variables such as family history and pain are not acceptable as the sole criteria for hysterectomy decisions for cis women patients. For cis women, family history is irrelevant to removing the cervix, for example, because the vast majority of cervical cancers cannot be explained by family history and are the result of the human papilloma virus. Cancer risk is also not a reliable indicator that hysterectomy should be pursued, at least not immediately. The BRCA-positive cisgender women in this study universally explained that after they had tested positive, their medical team suggested waiting to obtain a hysterectomy, despite their increased risk for developing uterine and ovarian cancers. The key consideration underlying this recommendation was the assumption that women necessarily want to become pregnant. Thus, hysterectomy was delayed for BRCA-positive cis women even though they, unlike many trans men in this study, had a documented increased risk of developing gynecological cancers. The notion that trans men might want to bear children is rarely considered unless the patient asks his physician about it.[3]

The experiences described by the trans men are particularly significant when compared to the standards of care in place for cisgender women. Although hysterectomies are the second most common surgery performed on individuals with internal reproductive organs, the standards of care have shifted in recent years to make these surgeries more dependent on clinical evidence (Temkin and Koh 2014). Like some trans men, some cis women are deeply physically and emotionally uncomfortable with pelvic exams and Pap tests, yet they are not given the same option for surgery as are trans men; nor can cis women typically access a hysterectomy due to an expression of pain (Bates, Carroll, and Potter 2011; Seymore et al. 1986). No matter how anxious or physically uncomfortable a cis woman may be, the surgical removal of organs is not seen by physicians as a medically appropriate alternative unless there is also a documentable finding upon clinical evaluation. Such findings could include fibroids, endometriosis (not family history but physical evidence of the condition), pelvic support problems, abnormal uterine bleeding, chronic pelvic pain (plus additional tests to ensure that hysterectomy is the best clinical decision), or gynecological cancer. Proceeding from these findings, clinicians embark on a series of tests and questions to ensure that hysterectomy is the best (and only) clinical decision for relieving pain (ACOG 2017; Lefebvre et al. 2002).

The recommendation that trans men have hysterectomies if they find gynecological exams uncomfortable represents a medical double standard and illustrates the degree to which expectations about gendered bodies shape standards of care independent of scientific evidence and patient desire. The ease with which trans men are presented with the option of a hysterectomy by medical providers is deeply embedded in cultural ideologies of gender. When women are faced with hysterectomies, they are confronted with what the surgery will mean for their femininity (see Elson 2004; Hallowell and Lawton 2002).

According to Jean Elson (2004), women who have hysterectomies find themselves in a liminal state between woman and not-woman. Often, the removal of these purportedly female organs and the resultant unsettling of gender identity occurs simultaneously with a loss of trust in medical authority. Gender identity is tied up in a struggle for bodily control between medical practitioners and patients, particularly when it comes to female reproductive organs. In their study of hysterectomy, Nina Hallowell and Julia Lawton found that women who have hysterectomies frequently express fears of physical masculinization (body changes, growth of facial hair, balding, deepening of voice) even though such an outcome is not scientifically supported (2002, 433). Women, in other words, did not fear losing their femininity (the dominant discourse used to explain the experience of gender-specific cancers). Instead, they feared impending masculinization but felt that controlling future risk far outweighed this concern.

The accounts presented by Hallowell and Lawton could suggest resistance to the dominant narratives of femininity and cancer. This logic is precisely what underlies the medical recommendation to offer hysterectomy to trans patients under circumstances that would not otherwise apply to cisgender women. Hysterectomy is culturally understood as a surgery that disrupts femininity. Although it is not a scientific fact (i.e., not evidence-based medicine), this cultural logic permeates the medical experiences of trans men.

The medical standard suggesting trans men and their providers consider hysterectomy may seem self-explanatory until one considers that this is not an option for cis women. If ovaries and uteri are merely body parts, then the identity of the patient should be irrelevant to clinical decision-making. Or if exams produce anxiety detrimental enough to prevent a person from seeking preventative care such as Pap tests, then hysterectomy should be a legitimate option for any person with these parts, regardless of that person's gender identity. That is, in terms of evidence-based medicine, either there is a scientific rationale for the surgery or there is not. If the principle of patient-centered care is being considered, then cis women should also have the option of a hysterectomy.

One complicating factor here is the role of hormones. Although not explicit, the recommendation that trans men undergo hysterectomies presupposes that these men are being treated with testosterone as part of their transition process. One of the key functions of the ovaries is producing estrogen. Removing these organs generally requires external hormone supplementation. For cis women, this would be estrogen replacement therapy; for trans men, testosterone is the protocol. Estrogen replacement therapy for women, particularly premenopausal women, is not medically advised. The use of testosterone by trans men has been accepted by the medical profession, however, thus rendering hysterectomies unproblematic.

The matter of hormones reinforces the point that removing currently healthy ovaries and uteri from trans men is unproblematic *because they are men*. Removing organs associated with women's bodies and femininity presumably brings the bodies of trans men into better alignment with their identities. However, the trans men I interviewed largely explained that these reproductive organs were inconsequential to their gender identities. Their perspective conflicts with the underlying medical assumption that ovaries and uteri have a greater gendered meaning.

It is important to recognize that transgender men have very different understandings of their reproductive organs. Some, like Kevin and Joe, are happy to be rid of their internal reproductive organs, regardless of whether they desire any surgical alteration of their external genitalia. Others may be interested in becoming pregnant, a desire that Noah felt the gynecologists he had seen could not understand. He stated that his questions about pregnancy and his potential to breastfeed "definitely cause confusion and providers either don't follow up or there's like this real weird curiosity." Noah also told me, "No one really knows what to do with most of my questions. People are definitely confused, and it doesn't line up with the storyline of what they think a trans guy should want or do."

When it comes to gynecological care, trans men occupy a difficult position. Providers and patients may expect—and many experience—discomfort during the exam. Dissociating is one possible strategy for managing discomfort. The stress of the exam may produce dissociative outcomes, including unconscious or intentional compartmentalization. Further, dissociation is connected to medical recommendations that trans men have hysterectomies rather than experience gynecological care. Underlying this stress is not necessarily discrimination or prejudice but a sense that gynecological care is the province of women. To be a man or to treat a man in this context is unthinkable, so trans patients and the medical profession must find strategies for managing this interactional crisis. While dissociating either with parts of the body or with the exam in its entirety is one approach, another oft-employed strategy is to embrace the role of the biocitizen through assertiveness: making one's needs and desires as a patient clear to health care providers.

The recommendation by the medical community that hysterectomy is a reasonable option for the prevention of gynecological cancer in trans men illustrates the degree to which expectations about gendered bodies and assumptions about patient desires shape standards of care independent of scientific evidence. For trans men, the path to hysterectomy is straightforward because of the way that gender operates as biopower: hysterectomy becomes a technology of power in the service of reproducing normative forms of gendered biolegitimacy. If the patient is uncomfortable or the insurance company will cover the surgery, then hysterectomy becomes a reasonable choice. However, this is not necessarily patient-centered care—hysterectomies attend as much to provider discomfort as patient discomfort. Without internal reproductive organs, there is no need for trans men to seek gynecological care thus shielding both patient and provider (although I argue it is largely the provider) from an uncomfortable clinical interaction.

The simplest resolution to awkward clinical interactions and the wrong body problem is to remove the offending organs and to bring patient bodies in closer alignment with the gender identity, based on normative cultural expectations. Removing these body parts is unremarkable because hysterectomy supposedly brings the body into greater alignment with gender identity, and providers tend to assume that the removal of organs associated with being female will improve the gender identity of their patients. Certainly, there are trans men who actively choose hysterectomies as part of their process of achieving gendered biolegitimacy, but it is detrimental to assume that this is appropriate, necessary, or desirable for all trans men. The men in this study rarely paid much attention to their reproductive organs, other than vague concerns about disease and death; they explained that these reproductive organs were inconsequential to their gender identities—thus conflicting with the underlying assumption that these organs have a greater gendered meaning.

The experiences of and standards of care for transgender men compared to the standards of care for cisgender women with respect to hysterectomy show that evidence-based medicine and patient-centered care cannot explain the different decision processes for these patient groups. The greater acceptance of hysterectomy as a response to patient anxiety about pelvic exams and Pap tests is understandable given expectations about what men's and women's bodies should be. The hysterectomy case suggests that removal of a healthy organ is shaped by ideas about men's bodies; in the case of trans men, hysterectomy can be deemed an acceptable risk because trans men are men. The case of bilateral mastectomies and breast reconstruction for cisgender women shows how such expectations play out for female bodies and why the removal of healthy body parts is medically justified in some cases but not in others.

Bilateral Mastectomy

The rate of elective prophylactic mastectomies has risen steadily for more than a decade, and they are in increasing demand as a preventive breast cancer measure (Grimmer et al. 2015; Hawley, Jagsi, and Marrow 2014; Tracy et al. 2013; Tuttle et al. 2007; Zeichner et al. 2014). This surgical technique is characterized by the removal of both healthy breasts (bilateral prophylactic mastectomy) or by the removal of the remaining healthy breast after a breast cancer diagnosis (contralateral prophylactic mastectomies). Part of the rise in prophylactic mastectomy rates is due to the increased availability of genetic testing for BRCA mutations and a growing medical consensus that prophylactic mastectomy is an appropriate response to a positive BRCA test. Although bilateral prophylactic mastectomies have become an increasingly accepted form of treatment for BRCA-positive women, contralateral prophylactic mastectomies remain highly contested. Ostensibly, bilateral and contralateral prophylactic mastectomies are the same surgical procedure: the removal of healthy breast tissue for the prevention of a future incidence of breast cancer. Yet the experience of accessing prophylactic mastectomy differs greatly for BRCA-positive women and women with breast cancer.

American medical practitioners generally reject the removal of healthy tissue unless there is a statistically significant risk of that tissue becoming diseased over time (as is the case with BRCA) because increased surveillance is understood to be a strong alternative for managing this increased risk. From this perspective, contralateral prophylactic mastectomies are unnecessary because these surgeries do not reduce breast cancer risk (Hawley, Jagsi, and Marrow 2014; Jin 2013; Katz and Morrow 2013; Rosenberg and Partridge 2014). Unless cancer is present in both breasts, physicians will not typically recommend a bilateral mastectomy, and some refuse outright to perform prophylactic mastectomies. Instead, providers will advocate for the removal of the diseased breast while leaving the healthy breast intact.

Despite these reservations, many breast surgeons will perform prophylactic mastectomies for women diagnosed with breast cancer, as evidenced by the number of women I spoke with who had had the procedure done. One study of contralateral prophylactic mastectomy argued that surgeons may be prone to "acquiesce to a patient's preference for more aggressive treatment" because they fear "adverse consequences in their practice"—such as losing the patient to another practice or decreased overall practice volume (Katz and Morrow 2013, 794). Other medical studies have suggested that, although patients claim that their decisions about prophylactic mastectomies stem from a desire to minimize risk and maximize quality of life, the appropriate course of action for physicians is to provide greater counseling in order to decrease rates of this surgery (Hawley, Jagsi, and Marrow 2014; Jin 2013; Katz and Morrow 2013; Morrow et al. 2014; Rosenberg and Partridge 2014). According to these physicians, providers are obliged to provide better information about the risks of prophylactic mastectomies and to mitigate the fact that "anxiety and fear certainly hamper optimal decision-making" (Rosenberg and Partridge 2014, 589).

At best, the medical community remains hesitant about prophylactic mastectomies even though patients overwhelmingly report a positive reaction to the surgery, with as many as 90 percent in one study claiming that they would make the same decision again (Jin 2013, 1548). The research that has suggested cis women are pleased with these decisions is often critiqued on the grounds that such claims about patient quality of life after prophylactic mastectomy "cannot be tested because patients cannot be randomized to the surgery" (Katz and Morrow 2013, 794). The position of the medical community is essentially that bilateral mastectomy does not significantly decrease risk of a second primary breast cancer and patient statements about quality of life cannot be trusted.

Of all the women with breast cancer I interviewed, only one spoke of a physician who brought up bilateral mastectomy. Colleen told me that she had asked her oncologist about mastectomy and her interest was brushed off. During the course of her treatment, Colleen's initial oncologist left for another position, and Colleen was referred to a different oncologist.

> [The new oncologist] actually brought mastectomy up when I met with her for the first time. She said, "Have you ever considered it?" And I said, "Yeah, I've actually considered it a lot." [The new oncologist] was, like, "I would do it. If I was in your position, I would do it in a heartbeat." And that was, like, sort of the validation that, you know, that—that kind of gave me the okay to say, like, all right, let's do it, because I've wanted to do this for eight years and having, you know, there's so much you're telling me now, yeah, that's totally appropriate, you're not crazy, you're not overreacting.

Although biomedical research suggests that mastectomy is an overused treatment for breast cancer, studies also indicate that women who choose this surgery are largely happy with their decision (see, for example, Frost et al. 2000). Thus, women with breast cancer and biomedical researchers stand in conflict over the appropriateness of bilateral mastectomies.

In chapter 2, the stories of women who chose bilateral mastectomy made clear that their decisions were largely based on their assessment of how various treatment plans would impact their health and quality of life. The experiences of women who have chosen prophylactic mastectomy and the assertions of medical researchers that these experiences do not constitute suitable data suggest a fundamental conflict between the medical principles of evidence-based medicine and patient-centered care. Patient-centered care suggests that patients' statements should be trusted and should have a strong impact on care; yet evidence-based medicine fundamentally discounts the credibility of patient-provided narratives about the impact of various treatments on quality of life unless those narratives match the assumptions about gendered bodies.

Stemming from the concept of doing no harm, as memorialized in the Hippocratic Oath, prevailing medical wisdom indicates that the removal of health tissue is inappropriate unless there is a significant statistical risk of disease over time, so increased surveillance is understood to be a strong alternative for managing an increased risk. The heightened risk of breast cancer due to a BRCA mutation has led to a gradually increased acceptance among medical professionals of prophylactic mastectomy. As a preventive measure, contralateral prophylactic mastectomies are far more contested than are bilateral prophylactic mastectomies, even though there may be an increased risk of developing a second cancer in the other breast.

As discussed in chapter 2, risk management is a significant decision-making framework for cisgender women diagnosed with breast cancer or a BRCA mutation. For these women, risk management is intrinsically connected to quality of life: the sense of normality that comes with forgoing increased screening and avoiding cancer. With respect to decisions about prophylactic mastectomy for women who are BRCA positive, health statistics have made prophylactic mastectomy a foregone conclusion. Women in the general U.S. population have about a 12 percent lifetime risk of breast cancer (National Cancer Institute 2018). Studies vary as to the exact lifetime risk for women with BRCA mutations, but researchers assess the risk as significantly higher than that of the general population, ranging from 45 percent to 82 percent depending on the type of BRCA mutation and ethnic heritage (Antoniou et al. 2003; Chen and Parmigiani 2007, King et al. 2003; National Cancer Institute 2018). In addition to BRCA there are a range of other genetic conditions and medical conditions that increase a woman's risk for breast cancer, which can influence her physician's surgical recommendations.

These statistical data are also important to patients in their decision-making process. No participant in this study who was diagnosed with a BRCA mutation reported that a physician tried to convince her not to have prophylactic mastectomies. The narrative of risk management is shared by patients and medical professionals with respect to BRCA diagnoses. Yet women diagnosed with breast cancer have had less success in using a risk management narrative to convince their health care providers of the merits of prophylactic mastectomy.

Currently, biomedical research does not support the notion that surgery significantly impacts a woman's survival rate after a breast cancer diagnosis unless she is at very high risk of developing cancer in her other breast. Instead, this research argues that increased surveillance is sufficient for mitigating risk of recurrence and that a desire for a bilateral mastectomy has more to do with an interest in the aesthetic outcome of breast reconstruction (Hawley, Jagsi, and

Marrow 2014; Jin 2013; Katz and Morrow 2013; Morrow et al. 2014; Rosenberg and Partridge 2014). However, increased surveillance is a hotly contested topic among medical professionals. Not only are the guidelines for screening frequency and timing debated, but so is the utility of these methods in actually preventing cancer (see Elmore et al. 2015; Kerlikowske et al. 2013). Women who chose bilateral mastectomy felt that the scientific uncertainty and emotional turmoil of the tests were more discomfiting than removing their breasts. The risk frame takes on different qualities based on provider perceptions of risk and quality of life. The participants in this study indicated that risk and quality of life have very different meanings for them than what were communicated by providers.

As described in chapter 2, women with breast cancer understood risk in terms of constant anxiety about increased frequency of screenings, recurrence, treatment complications, and the impact of these factors on loved ones. Linda, for example, was given the option to have a lumpectomy and radiation or a mastectomy. In contemplating her options, Linda was concerned about the effects of radiation and wary of a second cancer in her other breast. Suzy was also concerned about radiation because in the event of a recurrence the same area cannot be radiated again. Suzy felt that a mastectomy was an almost inevitable outcome and she might as well hedge her bets and remove both breasts.

The lack of a clear course of treatment, which Linda experienced, is not uncommon and can greatly contribute to a woman's decision to pursue bilateral mastectomy. Alison recalled that her breast surgeon "initially wasn't sure if a lumpectomy would be adequate." The range of medical options and the occasional difficulty in assessing the full extent of breast cancer can create what seems to patients to be considerable ambivalence about the most effective treatments. What women with breast cancer in this study tended to express was their feeling that a mastectomy, either unilateral or bilateral, was the surest means to prevent future risk of recurrence or a new diagnosis in the other breast.

Despite these patient concerns, physicians focused solely on the evidence of risk of cancer in the other breast and on the assumption that a desire for bilateral mastectomy was only related to a concern about the outcomes of reconstructive surgery. That is, the physicians focused on the current health of the specific body part under consideration. Edie was told by her physician, "No, I won't [perform contralateral prophylactic mastectomy] because there's nothing wrong with the other one. It's healthy. I'll send you for extra testing to make sure, but I'm certain it's benign, and I refuse to cut off a healthy body part." So Edie sought a second opinion and found a surgeon willing to do the procedure if that was her choice. Her first surgeon relied on the medical narrative of risk:

because the surgeon believed that the healthy breast was unlikely to develop cancer, he refused to perform the surgery. But for Edie the potential for cancer and the emotional risks associated with surveillance were too great *not* to have a bilateral mastectomy. Breast cancer patients insist that their fears about recurrence, treatment side effects, and the emotional trauma of surveillance detract from their overall quality of life and that bilateral mastectomy is their best option to protect their peace of mind.

The medical community is ambivalent about the risks and merits of elective prophylactic mastectomies. After her breast cancer diagnosis, Rachel's doctors tried to steer her away from a mastectomy. Her doctors told her, "You don't need to do that. We don't like the idea of doing that, but if it's your wish we will do it." She added, "The response was 'It's not necessary. You have a small early stage breast cancer. It's not necessary.'" Several participants disclosed their surgeons' reluctance when they broached the subject of prophylactic mastectomies. Colleen's surgeon urged caution in making this decision. "I had brought up mastectomy to my surgeon a few times, and her position was, 'I understand why you're interested in this, but it's not really necessary. I'm not going to talk you out of it if it's something you really want to do, but I want you to think about it.'" Women commonly described their surgeon's response in these terms. Physicians are basing their recommendations on data from medical studies suggesting that prophylactic mastectomies do not significantly reduce cancer risk, but many women want the surgery anyway.

Within the medical community, the risk of surgical complications also factors into recommendations for or against elective surgeries. In their comprehensive review of clinical studies of patients who had unilateral mastectomies compared with patients who had prophylactic bilateral mastectomies, Fahima Osman and colleagues (2013) indicate that women who have bilateral mastectomies have higher complication rates than women who have unilateral mastectomies. However, these complication rates remain low without reconstruction (7.6 percent); the higher rates of complications (64 percent) are associated with immediate reconstruction. Given that the participants in this study who chose bilateral mastectomies after breast cancer diagnoses desired to live flat, the complication rate was insufficient evidence to avoid surgery.

For women with breast cancer, the medical focus is on preserving a currently healthy body part—a consideration that apparently does not apply equally to transgender men or BRCA-positive cisgender women. The path to a mastectomy is fairly straightforward for a cisgender woman with a BRCA mutation. Although there remains some controversy, the medical community generally accepts that this surgery fits into the preventive health care model and can lead to a significant reduction in breast cancer risk. Although surveillance is an option for both BRCA-positive women and women with breast cancer, it is the only medically justifiable option recommended for women with breast cancer, even though these women are at increased risk (compared with the general population) for contralateral cancer. In the case of transgender men, the surgical recommendations do not focus on retaining healthy body parts but on ensuring that the bodies match the physical expectations for individuals with a given gender identity.

Medical risk is a critical consideration in decisions about elective surgeries to prophylactically remove a body part. For trans men and BRCA-positive cis women, this removal is warranted, yet for cis women with breast cancer it is not, based on an understanding of cancer risk. Bilateral mastectomies for cis women are implicitly understood as the removal of a body part essential to an identity as a woman. In the case of BRCA-positive women, this is justifiable because their cancer risk is so great. In addition, once removed, breasts can be surgically reconstructed to help restore that identity.

The medical community defines risks only in terms of medical outcomes, but the women I interviewed included emotional risks in their decision-making. Physicians are not uniformly averse to making surgical decisions based on patient anxiety, however. As I explained earlier in this chapter, standards of gynecological care for transgender men suggest that if patient anxiety about the gynecological examinations is too great, a hysterectomy is warranted; even a perfectly healthy and functional organ may be removed for the sole purpose of diminishing emotional strain that prevents an individual from seeking care. Such a surgery also continues to alter the patient's body in a way that aligns with the patient's gender identity—a trans male body without a uterus is comprehensible to the medical community. Cisgender women who identify as women and who wish to remove their breasts are unintelligible for some physicians. Both trans men and cis women in these instances are asking doctors to remove healthy tissue. It is unclear whether cis women may also avoid gynecological screenings out of anxiety, thus the extent of emotional upheaval may be invisible to medical providers. Aside from the visibility of anxiety, the key difference lies in the perception of patient gender.

As shown by participant narratives, women who choose to remove their breasts without clear medical evidence are often unintelligible. They challenge the commonly held belief that women have breasts. This reliance on evidence discounts the few qualitative studies that do exist and have been published in medical journals that find that women who choose contralateral mastectomies after a breast cancer diagnosis are quite happy with their decisions and would make the same decision again. Yet these data and the claims of patients are not always trusted by physicians. The women I interviewed who chose bilateral mastectomies after breast cancer diagnoses were often doubly confounding for physicians: they not only wanted to remove their breasts against the findings of biomedical research, but the majority also did not want to pursue breast reconstruction, a topic of great concern among plastic surgeons.

Breast Reconstruction

After mastectomy, many women choose not to undergo breast reconstruction. The percentage of women who do not obtain breast reconstruction ranges from 41.6 percent (Morrow et al. 2014) to 83.5 percent (Alderman et al. 2006).[4] Medical professionals are particularly concerned with these statistics because breast reconstruction is viewed as a critical component of positive psychological recovery because of its purported positive impact in helping patients cope with the loss of femininity, mood disturbances, and interpersonal, sexual, and marital dysfunction that can follow mastectomies (see, for example, Dean, Chetty, and Forrest 1983; Nahabedian 2020; Parker 2004; Rabinowitz 2013; Stavrou et al. 2009). In one prominent study, medical researchers found that "both immediate and delayed breast reconstructions provide substantial psycho-social benefits for mastectomy patients" and argued that "breast reconstruction may constitute a 'reverse mastectomy' offering the most effective means for restoring psychological wellbeing after a mastectomy" (Wilkins et al. 2000).

One commentary on this research within the medical community directly addresses these cultural beliefs: "The study [by Wilkins et al.] confirms much of what we know and *intuitively feel* about post-mastectomy breast reconstruction" (Cunningham 2000, 1026, emphasis mine). The statement "intuitively feel" is a signal that at the heart of biomedical interest in breast reconstruction are normative expectations about gendered bodies. This is not lost on those who choose breast reconstruction. Emily (BRCA positive) told me, "It really does come down to the fact that society defines a woman as a human who has breasts. And I think it's kind of like subconscious wiring of, well, I am a woman, and a woman must have breasts, so if I don't have breasts, I'm not a woman."

Although most studies of breast reconstruction espouse this belief, the work of Rowland et al. (2000) provides a dissenting view that women who have only mastectomies and women who have mastectomies with reconstruction do not report significant differences in body image or feelings of attractiveness. The critical difference here is that the Rowland study compared women who had reconstructive surgery with those who did not. Data from one group of patients without comparison simply indicates that those who had the surgery were content with their choice, not that making a different choice necessarily leads to a more negative outcome. Nor does it account for the many factors that can influence the effect this decision has on interpersonal, sexual, or marital dysfunction. The strength of ideologies of gender and sexuality are so great that studies like that by Rowland and colleagues, which run counter to commonsense assumptions, have little impact.

It is important to note that the American Board of Plastic Surgery classifies breast reconstruction as "reconstructive" as opposed to "cosmetic" surgery (2016). Cosmetic surgery is considered elective and aesthetic, whereas reconstructive surgery includes procedures that "restore or improve physical function and minimize disfigurement" (Dull and West 1991, 54). The emphasis on function and disfigurement is important in the context of breast cancer. The function of breasts cannot be repaired through reconstruction, and the form of the breast may also be somewhat compromised. What is chiefly restored through plastic surgery is the function of the breasts as visual markers of female identity in social interactions. This is what the medical community means by recovery.

Central to the biomedical framing of breast reconstruction is the idea that patients will have breast reconstruction if offered the option and are provided with examples of how successful the surgery can be. Patients are provided with formal information about reconstructive options, and physicians also told those I interviewed that reconstruction is "the fun part" of breast cancer. Katie's doctor told her, "You get a mastectomy, you get new breasts, and you get a tummy tuck. Which, post-children sounded like a great idea to me."

Many women find great pleasure in being breasted, and breast reconstruction can be central to restoring a sense of self after the physical and emotional difficulties of breast cancer. When faced with the possibility of mastectomies, many of the women I interviewed turned to the internet to search for images of both reconstructed breasts and flat, postmastectomy chests because medical providers failed to offer information about living flat. After seeing these images and understanding the specifics of breast reconstruction as presented by physicians, several women expressed sentiments similar to, but not always as colorful as, Edie. Her response to reconstructive surgery after viewing images on the internet was, "Not on my fucking life!"

Despite their desire and informed intent to live flat, the women I interviewed reported that physicians made great efforts to convince them to have surgery. Fran had to watch a video extolling the benefits of reconstruction before making her final decisions. She found the video offensive: "It was infuriating to me after having made the decision [to live flat] to have this tape that seemed to imply that I had made the wrong decision because all these people were so happy. And I was now going to be unhappy for the rest of my life."

Catherine had to undergo expensive psychological testing when she told her doctor that she wanted to live flat. "My doctors were kind of floored that I would want to spend the rest of my life without reconstruction, and I felt as though they kept on pushing it throughout my entire chemotherapy experience. . . . It was a constant questioning of my mental state and my decision-making process." She was required to undergo psychological screenings with approved providers not covered by her insurance. Linda's doctor asked her simply, "Do you want to be mutilated?"

In other cases, there was no discussion between patient and provider. Some women, like Suzy, assumed that a flat chest is the default result of a mastectomy. She explained, "I never mentioned it to him because I figured, well, I'm not having reconstruction, why should I bring it up? Six weeks after the surgery, I was still very lumpy, and I asked him about that, and he says, 'Oh, you know, that's the excess skin so that you can get an implant later.' . . . The fact that this man assumed that I wanted to have this done, and left skin that I didn't want, has been quite distressing for me." Despite her desire to live flat, Linda's surgeon left skin that she described as "sharp points and looking down they look like shirt collars. They had substance to them, like cartilage." For both Linda and Suzy, their surgeons assumed that they would eventually want breast reconstruction and purposefully left extra skin to accommodate implants, even though neither woman had expressed this interest to her physician.

Each of these stories involves the element of time between diagnosis and surgery. For some women, there is time to research options about mastectomy and reconstruction. They are then able to make an informed decision about their options. When there is less time to investigate and consider options, women must often make decisions about breast reconstruction at the same time as mastectomy. This compressed timetable often leads to privileging the biomedical imaginary of women's bodies over women's own desires.

The window between diagnosis and surgical treatment can range from one week to several months. The timeline is determined by medical providers through assessment of a patient's diagnosis. Physicians expect women with a breast cancer diagnosis to process a significant amount of information in a short period of time. A week or two is very little time with which to deal with the emotional and logistical realities of this diagnosis. Breast reconstruction often begins immediately after mastectomy, with the placement of expanders so long as the patient is not beginning radiation. As a result, breast reconstruction can seem to be a normal part of the mastectomy process.

Kate got swept up in this process and didn't give reconstruction much consideration. "There was lots going on. Nobody's really telling me I need to get reconstructed at all, it's just you can get it. So, you kind of think, well, if they're taking things away, I should have them replaced." When Kate later developed an infection and physicians determined she could not continue with reconstruction until after radiation, she had time to research and consider what it really meant to have reconstruction. As a staunch feminist, she found herself surprised that she had opted for reconstruction in the first place. When Kate had time to focus on her options in the absence of the pressure that her diagnosis originally brought, she decided that living flat was the best choice for her in terms of both her health and her politics.

Samantha took three months after her prophylactic mastectomy to decide whether to reconstruct her breasts.

> I was offered reconstruction at the time, and I said no, I'm not sure I want to do that yet. And so about three months down the road when I went back to my medical oncologist, I said I'm done. No more surgeries. I'm fine with this. I don't feel the need to go back and have more surgery. And I'm grateful that you guys gave me that choice because so many women don't have the choice. . . . And so, in 2011 I had the first mastectomy. 2012 I had the second mastectomy. I finished the chemo in December of 2011, and in July or August of 2012 I went in and said, okay, I'm strong enough. Let's do this.

Her surgeons were unusual in that they presented living flat as an option. Samantha described her medical providers as a "dream team" who responded well to her "incessant need to know what's going on and to take time to decide what to do about reconstruction. Between her mastectomies, Samantha described herself as "uni-boob"—that is, she was flat on one side and often wore a prosthetic. After the prophylactic mastectomy, she briefly wore prosthetics and then tried living flat in public. This was an important time for Samantha as she determined what shape she wanted her body to have over time.

> I did it more because I was trying to see if I really needed to have breasts, you know, to wear clothing and stuff like that. Where was my comfort zone with not having breasts anymore? . . . [The prosthetics] kept sliding up to my chin. So I was constantly pulling them down. Finally, one day I thought, this is ridiculous. It's not comfortable, and I'm just going to try going without [the prosthetics] and see how I handle that emotionally. At first, I was self-conscious that other people would have a hard

> time with it. And then I quickly realized that, in my opinion, people didn't even notice. But it was a gradual process. I hadn't talked to anybody who had decided to stay flat. I'd only talked to women who had decided to have the reconstructive surgery. And I kept thinking, okay, that's their journey, but is it mine? And I thought, if I find in this process that a part of my self-image is connected to having breasts, and it's too emotionally hard for me, I'll go back and I'll have it done. But I need to try this out, too. And I have the option at any point in my future to go in for reconstruction. But right now, I'm totally okay with the way things are.

Time was thus crucial for Samantha. She was able to try out living with one breast, living with prosthetics, and living flat. Her medical team was able to give her the resources she needed to make her decision, including access to medical literature and time. When the time to make a decision about reconstruction is short, however, gender ideologies provide a shortcut for providers and patients in determining what course of action to take.

Edie also described the importance of time in influencing her decision about reconstruction. "Had we done the mastectomy right away, they probably would've put in the tissue expanders because I don't think I would've had enough time to really think it through or research pro and con, you see what I mean, because it was presented as this is just the way you do it." Many women knew what their reconstruction choice would be as soon as they realized breast cancer or BRCA was a likely diagnosis. For others, time was crucial because they had not considered what a breast cancer or BRCA diagnosis would mean for their embodied identity.

The time to research can have drastically different impacts on women with breast cancer and women with BRCA mutations. Women with breast cancer typically have little time to consider options because the imperative to treat the disease before it can metastasize is so strong. Women with a BRCA diagnosis and no breast cancer can wait for years to decide whether to have a prophylactic mastectomy and how to reconstruct the body afterward. Julie, for example, received her BRCA test results fifteen months before our interview in October, and she had a prophylactic mastectomy planned for the following summer. For over two years Julie had contemplated the impact of mastectomy and reconstruction on her life. She spent much of this time researching the various types of reconstruction options and determined that a version of the TRAM (transverse rectus abdominis muscle) flap procedure was the best choice for her: "I have done a lot of research on reconstruction. It's terribly imperfect, [and] I don't think that I'm going to come out of it looking the way I look now and that's difficult to accept. I've been doing a lot of research about what gets the best cosmetic results, and it seems like using your own tissue, it does produce the best cosmetic results."

For Samantha, time to research proved essential because she needed to process the emotional consequences of her diagnosis, the treatment options of surveillance versus prophylactic mastectomy, and the various available forms of reconstruction. Samantha represents an extreme among the BRCA positive women I interviewed, but the process she was in the midst of at the time of our interview represents that undertaken by many women. Many BRCA women had time before pursuing genetic testing to consider their options in the event of a positive diagnosis because family members had also tested positive. Seeing close relatives grapple with the process and taking time to decide whether to pursue testing gave BRCA-positive women additional time to consider reconstruction before receiving test results.

The amount of time women have to think through their options is largely determined through medical interactions. In these interactions, physicians have the power to determine the treatment timeline and to assess the risks associated with delaying decision-making. In this way, the element of time can affect patients' ability to fulfill the obligations of biocitizenship—that is, to research and make an informed decision about their health.

Living flat is rarely an option presented to women, even when time is not a critical issue. A pamphlet provided to cisgender women at one prominent cancer treatment facility anticipates questions a patient may have as she considers breast reconstruction, including "Do I have to have breast reconstruction?" Although the answer in the pamphlet is "no," the response mostly concerns breast prostheses and concludes with these two sentences: "Living a long cancer-free life is our goal. Keeping your femininity is just as important, too" (Crosby 2010). Regardless of how much time a woman has to research options, ideologies of gendered embodiment serve as shortcuts in the decision-making process.

For some women, breasts are integral to their identities as feminine women, yet participants who live flat challenged the association of breasts with femininity. Samantha stated that, after her contralateral mastectomy without reconstruction, "I feel more feminine than I've ever felt." In this respect, a sense of embodied femininity can be important both for those who choose reconstruction and those who live flat. Samantha and other women like her highlight the taken for granted connection between breasts and femininity and suggest that femininity can be embodied in other ways.

The risk narrative also plays into some women's decisions about reconstruction. Concern about postsurgical complications is a factor in some women's decision to avoid reconstruction or to reverse the surgery after it had been done. Depending on the type of reconstruction and individual health factors, reconstructive surgeries can have a complication rate of up to 46.4 percent (see Brooke, Mesa, and Uluer 2012; Jagsi et al. 2014; Sullivan et al. 2008). Alison explained that "the things [the surgeon] was telling me didn't really correspond with what I had read about the complications that reconstruction surgery can bring about, the length of the process, you know, how many procedures it takes." Instead, the surgeon emphasized reconstructive surgery as "the fun part" of having breast cancer. Another participant, Kate, developed a serious infection in her implant and ultimately decided to have the surgery reversed. Despite the very real risks of complication and poor evidence suggesting a strong correlation between surgery and positive experiences in recovery, reconstruction is an elective surgery that physicians advocate for strongly in interactions with patients.

Breast reconstruction is also not an option routinely presented to men with breast cancer. Due to having less breast tissue than the average cisgender woman, men diagnosed with breast cancer typically only have mastectomy as a surgical treatment option. Frank paraphrased his surgeon's opinion on the matter, stating, "You're a guy. It's a rather simple decision." Many men in this study reiterated that a mastectomy is an easier decision for men than for women. Ezra explained that "going through a single or double mastectomy affects [women] a lot more psychologically because it is so wrapped up with your image as a feminine person. For guys it's just an inconvenience . . . it's not that bad." In describing the mastectomy and recovery, Frank's surgeon told him, "We'll remove the breast and that will just be the end of it. For a woman, he said there'll be other issues, but they are usually not an issue for a man. That would be the end of the discussion." For men, there was no additional discussion of breast reconstruction as there would be for women.

Larry lamented the fact that breast reconstruction was not offered. His providers explained that reconstruction was available, but that men generally do not do it. Tim was the only cisgender man I interviewed who explicitly asked his medical team about reconstruction. After meeting with a plastic surgeon, he ultimately decided that the options of tattooing or nipple reconstruction were "weird." The lack of choice about reconstruction is significant, given the concerns men shared in this study regarding their postmastectomy bodies. Frank felt "deformed." Ed expressed his desire not to "cause people any queasiness." Ed described having a concave chest after surgery and expressed that he would have appreciated being offered something to fill the space.

Reconstruction is thus framed as necessary for healing, but only for women. This framing is not based on actual medical evidence, nor is it truly based on a concern for patient-centered care. Women who wanted to live flat were pressured to have reconstruction. Cisgender men were not offered reconstruction or felt ashamed for asking about it. This inconsistency highlights normative expectations about gendered bodies. Recovery from breast cancer, a disease that threatens gender identity, is only complete when these expectations are restored or preserved.

Conclusion

The accounts of elective surgery described in this chapter suggest that decisions about elective surgery in gynecological and breast cancer care are not primarily about medical evidence (specifically health risks) or patient-centered care. The experiences of cis women who live flat and trans men, when compared with those of cis women who reconstruct and cis men, suggest that decisions about cancer care for breast and gynecological cancers are not suitably explained through principles of evidence-based medicine or patient-centered care. Instead, these cases suggest that medical recommendations turn on shaping patient bodies in accordance with normative ideologies of gender.

Only those who shape their bodies through surgical means in accordance with gender norms receive official support from the medical establishment. Medical recommendations for different groups of patients have inherent contradictions that are best explained through an understanding of the taken-for-granted assumptions about men, women, and their respective bodies. These beliefs on the part of providers both influence the care patients receive and serve to reproduce ideologies of gender. Medical interactions are critical in the process of legitimating normative ideas about gendered bodies. If the gender problem in medicine is to be solved, medical professionals and social researchers need to collaborate to better understand the ways in which cultural ideologies shape clinical practice and, in turn, reproduce these ideologies.

The role of technology cannot be understated. One of the key means by which to build gendered biolegitimacy in moments of bodily disruption is through medical technology, whether it be medications, surgeries, or other therapeutic methods. There is a clear tension demonstrated by the cases described in this chapter. In the hands of medical professionals, these three surgeries can be technologies of power. As the participants explained, their experiences with physicians situated access to hysterectomies, prophylactic mastectomies, and breast reconstruction as technologies of power. That is, these interventions were deployed or withheld by medical professionals in order to shape the patients' bodies in accordance with normative expectations of gender. These same surgeries can also be understood as technologies of the self when desired by patients in order to shape their bodies in ways that reflect an authentic sense of identity. It is in resolving this tension that new forms of gendered biolegitimacy may emerge over time.

The medical interactions in this chapter focus on elective surgery, but I suspect that they are not unique contexts in which biomedical imaginaries of healthy embodiment coalesce with sociocultural imaginaries of gendered embodiment. These surgeries make visible the ways in which medical practitioners bring cultural ideologies into the examination room in ways that often go unnoticed. The exception is when individual patients have a different idea of what their personal medical outcome should be. The concept of doing gender—that is, making one's gender visible in social interactions in accordance with cultural norms—applies to medical interactions as well as the sorts of everyday interactions on which West and Zimmerman (1987) built their theory. Medical training does not remove the influence of the cultural ideologies that constantly shape individual perceptions of the world. Instead, the combination of evidence-based medicine and patient-centered care creates the illusion for health care providers that they are participants in objective science while allowing them to invoke normative gender expectations in the service of providing patient-centered care.

The underlying notion is that all people need to be socially intelligible and this intelligibility can be perceived through the body. This is the heart of gendered biolegitimacy. Due to their relative authority in a society marked by biopolitics, physicians wield an enormous power in determining legitimate and illegitimate bodies through their interactions with patients. Consequently, medical care is both shaped by ideas about gender and reproduces those beliefs through the bodies of patients, unless the patients themselves actively resist this process.

Conclusion

Gendered Biolegitimacy and the Medical Profession

Throughout this book I have argued that gender is problematic for medicine, but not in the way that might be readily apparent. Certainly, health disparities between and among men and women exist. Gender also remains influential in matters from physician–patient trust to the training of medical students and the specialties individuals choose (see, for example, Arnold, Martin, and Parker 1988; Risberg et al. 2003). As biomedical research has begun to attend to physiological differences between women and men, clinical practice has shifted to account for these differences in the diagnosis and treatment of disease. Yet gender is more than simply a variable impacting health distribution and professional composition. Instead, I have argued that medical practices are embedded within the gender system and as such are influenced by and reinforce commonly held beliefs about what it means to be a man or a woman. These beliefs are specifically tied to the physical body, and accordingly the authority of medical providers becomes critical in rendering legitimate and recognizable a patient's gender while at the same time reaffirming normative expectations for appropriately gendered bodies.

The cases presented in the preceding chapters point to ways in which individuals both affirm and resist norms of gender and health. Drawing on the imperatives of biocitizenship, these narratives of integrity and authenticity demonstrate the link between identity, embodiment, and the ability to be recognized as a whole person in daily interactions. It is this intersection of gender, identity, embodiment, and social recognition that gendered biolegitimacy attempts to encompass. Resistance becomes an embodied act as subjects negotiate health care and health behaviors. Understanding gender as biopower and patients as biocitizens creates an opportunity to imagine alternate embodiments and to advocate for the legitimacy of these embodiments. Although gender, as biopower, was initially created and legitimized by medical professionals, the meaning and value associated with gender are created through ongoing processes of interaction. The experiences people have outside the clinic shape their desires within it. In this way new meanings can influence clinical interactions, but doing so involves confronting biopower. Gendered biolegitimacy creates an opportunity to examine what gender means, how it shapes and is shaped by human bodies, and how some bodies become socially intelligible while acknowledging the key role that the medical profession plays in these processes.

Case Summary/Comparison

Medical care presumes a particular alignment of gender identity, body, and treatment. When these components are out of alignment, medical practitioners must alter some combination of the treatment plan, the treatment interaction, or the patient's body. When the misalignment is the result of a "natural accident," such as male breast cancer, practitioners may take steps to alter the treatment of and interaction with patients in order to preserve the normative alignment between identity and body. This approach was evident in the accounts of cisgender men whose interactions during the course of treatment revolved around "protecting" women patients from the presence of men in a clinical space defined by femininity and by normalizing men patients through the use of different colored gowns and language in order to affirm that men get breast cancer, too. Although they are also seeking care in woman-centered spaces, transgender men have had a markedly different experience than cis men. Trans men described their struggles with the bodily terminology and gynecological care that facilitated altering their bodies through hysterectomy. Rather than experiencing medical care that affirmed their identities as men, trans men generally experienced care that questioned their identities or problematized their bodies.

The comparison between cis women who live flat and those who choose breast reconstruction reflects similar patterns of medical scrutiny for those patients who choose to alter their bodies in ways that resist normative expectations for gendered bodies. Like cis men with breast cancer, cis women who are BRCA positive are seen as simply unlucky, and the role of the physician is to correct this misfortune through surgical interventions, chiefly mastectomy and breast reconstruction. The "accident" of a genetic anomaly (BRCA) and the standard treatment (bilateral prophylactic mastectomy) intervene in the expected alignment of patient identity and body. Because this treatment is considered medically necessary, the logical next step is to engage in an additional intervention to realign body and identity with ideologies about what a woman's body should be. Like trans men, cis women who choose prophylactic mastectomy against prevailing medical wisdom alter their bodies in ways that disrupt the expected identity-body-ideology relationship. When providers acquiesce, they expect and encourage women to have breast reconstruction. A patient's questioning of or rejecting this procedure may mark her as suspect and troublesome.

To be clear, these differences are not simply a matter of medical evidence or the objective assessment of medical risks. Often medical treatment is in opposition to medical evidence (such as recommendations for trans men to have hysterectomies simply because they are uncomfortable with gynecological examinations), is conducted without medical evidence (such as breast cancer treatments for cis men when all research has been conducted with cis women), or is supported by studies purporting to be objective but are actually heavily influenced by the status quo of gender (such as the greater evidentiary weight given to studies explaining the psychosocial benefits of breast reconstruction compared to studies reporting that flat women are just as satisfied after mastectomy). The cycle of care for breast and gynecological cancers (and potentially other illnesses) is ideally a balance between evidence-based medicine and patient-centered care. The experiences of cis women who live flat and trans men, compared with those of cis women who reconstruct and cis men, suggest, however, that decisions about cancer care for breast and gynecological cancers are not suitably explained through these principles. Instead, these cases show that providers' care decisions shape patient bodies in accordance with normative ideologies of gender. My research indicates that care decisions made by both patients and providers are largely shaped by commonly held beliefs about what it means to be a woman or a man and how those meanings map onto and shape the physical body. These beliefs, on the part of providers, shape gender. Gender is not a variable determining access to care and health outcomes, nor is it an individual attribute. Instead, medical practices are embedded within the gender system, and as such are influenced by cultural ideologies of gender. Medical care is both shaped by ideas about gender but also reproduces those beliefs through the bodies of patients.

Health and medical care are critical arenas for studying gender. Theoretical approaches to this topic must be able to account for gender as more than a category of difference because health has become central to American life. The idea of gendered biolegitimacy attempts to merge scholarship on biopolitics and biocitizenship with theories of gender and health. For both patients and medical providers, gender identity and health are intertwined. With the advent of gender-specific medicine, a better understanding of how medical care bolsters or threatens the gender structure is imperative to improving access and freedom of decision-making for patients.

That gender is problematic for medicine is not simply a matter of academic theorizing. The level of gatekeeping power the medical profession has over determining and legitimizing gender identity and gendered embodiment has real and intense consequences on whether trans, gender nonconforming, and (as shown in this book) cis people can live livable lives. This is a power that perhaps no professional group should exert, yet we live in a world where this is the reality. As such, the medical profession needs to acknowledge, address, and perhaps limit the exercise of these powers in order to truly listen to patients and to fulfill a professional obligation to "do no harm." That is, medical professionals need to learn to accept a patient's definition of harm and work within that definition rather than only rely on normative and patronizing assumptions about harm and quality of life.

It remains essential to bring ethnomethodological theories of gender to bear on clinical practice. This does not necessitate abandoning other research that employs gender as a binary category in order to better understand various therapeutic treatments and the trajectories of disease. Rather, this research must occur in a context that clearly delineates the situatedness of biomedical practice (both research and clinical care) within the gender system and other structures that lead to inequality. In addition, medical practitioners need to be trained in relational theories of gender with a clear explanation of how taken-for-granted gender ideologies shape clinical judgment and the power that health care providers have in maintaining or challenging structures of inequality through medical practice. This need presents an opportunity not just for sociologists to train health care providers but also for innovative collaborations between medical and social researchers to improve our understanding of the complexities of health care and the role of health care in maintaining (and potentially changing) the cultural system of gender. This research would also add rich empirical data to ongoing feminist engagement with gender, the body, and health.

Rethinking Medical Education

The stories shared in this book prompt a question: How do we change medical culture to be able to adapt to and respect the changing needs of the patient population? In some respects, the medical community is asking this question of themselves. In the following recommendations, I focus on physicians because this is the group that is at the top of the medical hierarchy in terms of decision-making power over patients. These recommendations could be adapted for nurses, physician assistants, and other types of health care providers. A wide variety of scholars have critiqued the expectation that Western science is necessarily objective and able to neutralize bias (see, for example, Harding 2004a, 2004b; Longino 1990). Following from this tradition, I implore the medical community to acknowledge and explore the cultural norms that influence and bias their treatment of patients as well as their role in upholding normative ideologies that routinely dismiss patients in a range of ways.

The addition of a sociology section to the Medical College Admission Test (MCAT) is an important move for the medical profession because it provides an opportunity to familiarize future physicians and other prehealth students with sociological concepts in ways that move beyond biomedical interest in cultural competence to encouraging serious grappling with medicine's embeddedness within the gender structure (indeed, within all systems of difference, including structures of race and class). These recent changes to the MCAT also have the potential to bring prehealth students into sociology classrooms, where in prior years these students may have had to prioritize physical and biological science courses to prepare for their chosen profession. There is an opportunity here to not only aid future medical students in passing a standardized test but help them begin to question the underlying assumptions of medicine and the embeddedness of the profession within systems of difference. This in turn can bring about eventual changes to the gender system.

Although the inclusion of social science in the MCAT is critical in establishing these fields as a real and recognizable component of medicine, more needs to be done. At the time of this writing, sociology, psychology, history, and philosophy are not systematically required coursework in pre-med or postbaccalaureate programs in the United States. Requiring that social science courses be part of pre-med curricula—particularly with respect to the social construction of race, gender, and sexuality; history and philosophy of science and medicine; and social psychology in particular—would provide an academic foundation to question some of the basic assumptions of the medical profession while giving future health care providers the tools to examine their own biases and normative assumptions about who patients are and what they actually desire. This would bring humanity back into the medical profession as a balance for the scientifically based training these students currently receive.

Including these courses at the undergraduate or postbaccalaureate level is necessary but insufficient. Medical schools must continue these courses at the graduate level and incorporate faculty with these research specialties into the medical school community. Another option would be to increase the number of fully funded joint MD-PhD programs with social science fields. According to the Association of American Medical Colleges (AAMC), there are one-hundred and twenty-five joint MD-PhD programs (2019a). Of these, thirty-two (25 percent) offer a joint degree with anthropology, history, history or sociology of science, philosophy, psychology, sociology, or gender studies. Eleven of these thirty-two (8 percent) offer sociology degrees, and two (1.6 percent) offer gender studies degrees (AAMC 2019b). Incorporating these fields into a standard medical education would allow physicians to more fully understand the relationship between medicine and social structures, rather than seeing medicine as merely an objective science that exists outside these structures. Additionally, such study would establish the socially constructed nature of medical knowledge and of the profession. This would provide a much needed counternarrative to the taken-for-granted assumptions about gender prevalent in our culture. The stories of participants presented throughout this work suggest that such assumptions are extremely detrimental to the well-being of patients.

Again, these changes are necessary but insufficient. Social science—not just social determinants of health, but the relationship between medicine and social structures—must also be included on all three "steps" of the U.S. Medical Licensing Examination (USMLE). As it currently stands, the three steps of the USMLE assess the scientific and clinical knowledge of future physicians. In order to pass medical school, receive a medical license, and move on to residency, future physicians must pass all three steps. Adding in social science as part of the requirements to receive a license reinforces and legitimizes the fact that physicians practice medicine within social structures and are influenced by the cultural assumptions embedded within those structures. Without attending to these norms, medicine will necessarily reinforce existing assumptions while obstructing those patients who seek to find alternate ways of being.

Finally, the process of board certification for physicians by specialty after completing residency requires ongoing assessment by the American Board of Medical Specialties. This is not part of maintaining a medical license; rather, these are standards set by the various subspecialties. Maintaining board certification requires meeting standards in core competencies. Adding a sociology or knowledge of social structures competency would create a foundation for ongoing engagement with social science scholarship. Maintaining a medical license requires completing a certain number of Continuing Medical Education (CME) credits. Social science–based CME credits need to be available and required for maintenance of a medical license.

Importantly, this call to incorporate social science at all levels of medical education and licensure needs to be developed through collaboration with social scientists. Social scientists must be included in the professional assessment of physicians based on these standards. To be clear, the culture of medicine needs to change in order to discontinue the blind reproduction of social norms that do not apply universally or equally across patient populations.

These broad implications of my research also suggest a specific avenue for future research within the context of female cancers. To provide a more nuanced understanding of gendered biolegitimacy, it will be necessary to explore provider narratives of care for the patient groups identified in my research. I have described *patient perceptions* of these encounters, an approach that prioritizes the lived experiences of those who must bear the consequences of medical decisions in their everyday lives. Investigating these scenarios with medical professionals will help identify the implicit and explicit processes by which ideologies of gender influence health care. In addition, a thorough investigation of these concepts in the context of medical education will identify those points throughout the physician curriculum where ideologies of gender can be brought from the margins to the center of physician education, thus promoting a necessary engagement with normative expectations for patient bodies while critically examining what is meant by health when treating patients.

Final Thoughts

Medicine is a social institution with important ramifications for the social structures that organize social life. Medical interactions require categorizing bodies as ill or healthy, normal or pathological, treatable or untreatable. Accordingly, the production of medical knowledge and the provision of health care are based on and reinforce definitions of normal bodies. Throughout this book, I have argued that this categorization, like most everyday interactions, begins with a determination of gender. The process of doing and determining gender within the medical context is especially fraught because bodies are explicitly on display in ways for which earlier theories of interaction are unable to account. Further, these medical interactions involve a process of legitimation whereby medical providers and patients are engaged in maintaining or resisting the gender system.

This system can be threatened in two ways. The first is by an "accident of nature" that alters the body. Such is the case for cisgender men diagnosed with breast cancer and cisgender women diagnosed with BRCA. Medical providers target their treatment plans not only to address illness and restore the body to a state of health, but also to restore the dignity of gender that these diagnoses imperil. The second threat to the system is through those patient choices perceived by physicians as willful disregard of normative treatment and normative expectations of gender. When transgender men follow medical advice and seek gynecological care, and when cisgender women elect to have contralateral prophylactic mastectomies after a breast cancer diagnosis and then choose to live flat, they confront a medical system that is confounded by them. Although their decisions are based in a desire to be healthy, these patients disrupt the alignment between identity, body, and gender ideologies upon which medical care relies. In order to move beyond the binary assessment of gender in biomedicine, we must dig deeper to understand how the system of gender operates on and through medical care.

What, then, is at stake in understanding the role of gender ideologies in medical care? This is not just a concern for gender and sexual minorities. Rather, because biocitizenship is predicated on our standing as women and men, the influence of gender ideologies (and gendered embodiment in particular) is central to the medical interactions every person has throughout their lifetime. Normative expectations about gendered embodiment, bodily practices, and identity shape medical care at its core; and the a priori (and instantaneous) categorization of patients determines what diagnoses and recommendations are made to patients. This system of care also suggests that values are critical in health care decisions. Typically, medical interactions do not value a holistic sense of the patient's well-being. Instead, these interactions privilege the status quo of gender, assumptions about who counts as a man or woman based on physical characteristics, and which bodies are valued in social life based on their assimilation into normative expectations of gender. This practice does not help patients or providers, nor do these values enhance whatever it is we mean by "health."

Gendered biolegitimacy is a way to understand how the way we value gender in society combines with biocitizenship and medical authority to render some patients socially visible and others invisible. Medical attempts to restore health by shaping patient's bodies and explaining treatment options in line with normative gender expectations reinforce these ideals. Accordingly, only certain relationships between bodies and identities become legitimate through biomedical interactions and authority. This is the heart of gendered biolegitimacy. Although medical providers have the greatest power in determining what counts as a legitimately gendered body, this process also occurs in daily interactions through the policing of bodies in locker rooms, at beaches or swimming pools, in the workplace, and at home. In other words, gendered biolegitimacy is a cyclic, interactive process that is reinforced not just in everyday life but also through interactions with medical authorities.

The last two decades have seen rapid shifts in the ability of trans and cis patients alike to access medical interventions that shape our bodies as we wish.

It is hard, however, to be hopeful after hearing the stories of individuals who felt that their desires and questions were dismissed by medical professionals and after reading medical scholarship that has uniformly discounted the kinds of stories told in this book. But there is an underlying strength and power in these stories. Although the clinic can feel like an isolating experience and patients may feel alone as they advocate for embodiments that feel right but have not acquired a wide degree of legitimacy, it is through the resistance and redefinition of meaning for which individual patients fight that change may occur. The more each patient advocates for themselves, the more difficult it will become for the medical profession to ignore the types of change that desires for alternative embodiments require.

Instead of optimism or despair, I offer this prognosis for the future: any change that may occur in the operation of biopower in the context of medicine will need to be a joint effort between patients and providers, with patients serving as the primary catalysts for change. In this final chapter, I have suggested ways forward for the medical community through real engagement with the wealth of social science scholarship on gender. But unless the imbalance of power in knowledge and decision-making authority between patients and providers is reconciled through intentional effort, the rate of change will be slow indeed. Gender matters, and the materiality of gender matters. These matter to patients and to providers. Medicine will need to play catch up for the foreseeable future to match the pace of change that gender-expansive people require.

I believe that the greatest obstacle to creating greater legitimacy for a variety of gendered embodiments comes from the physician's ethic to do no harm. What the stories told by participants in this project suggest is that "harm" must be defined by the patients, through processes of informed consent that include a greater range of sources that count as information: patients truly believe themselves to be authorities on their own lives and bodies, and want to assert this authority in all contexts. These are not new struggles, and the meanings and variety of expressions associated with gender will continue to evolve. It is the responsibility of the medical profession to evolve alongside them, to serve as supports for patients rather than as gatekeepers and obstacles to interventions that will improve the quality of life and therefor the health of all patients.

Appendix A

Methodological Note

This research began as I tried to make sense of two concurrent events: the gynecological issues of a transgender friend and a controversy over a homophobic e-mail sent out by a few students at a socially progressive medical school in the northeast United States. As I attended talks and workshops sponsored by the medical school and talked with medical students, I began to recognize that there is something uncomfortable about the relationship between the way medicine is practiced and the management of patient identity. I watched the ways that the structure of medical education worked to rebuild students as physicians—people distinct from and, in some ways, above lay people.

Despite providing some attention to cultural diversity and to ideas of holistic treatment, medical training was flawed in that the emphasis was on using these measures to increase patient compliance with medical advice. It was not about questioning the cultural assumptions that might influence care. In short, physical science ruled the medical curriculum, and any other training was marginal and subordinate to it. The training of physicians and the experiences of patients are often at odds in care.

The puzzle is this: who I am is more than my body, but it is also deeply my body. How patients and providers navigate this paradox is central to the adequacy of care that patients receive.

The Importance of Narrative

Storytelling is a key method for making sense of the world we live in. It is a way to build theory that resonates with everyday experience. I began each interview with a single prompt, asking each participant to imagine that they were about to write a novel, movie, or play about their experience with breast/gynecological cancer care. Then I asked them to describe the opening scene. From there, I listened and let the other person unravel the story. The power of narrative is well documented, particularly with respect to health experiences (see Charon 2006; Charon and Montello 2002; Charon and Wyer 2008; Childress 2002; Frank 1995, 2000; Williams 1984). When people tell their stories, they not only construct their identity, but in the case of this research they are also constructing the meaning of their bodies and presenting new possibilities of how gender can be embodied.

Central to my research design is the notion that cancer queers the body in the sense that gynecological and breast cancers have the effect of disrupting the stability of gender and sexuality not only for the person with the disease diagnosed but for all those around them, including their physicians. The stories the participants shared are queer in the sense that no matter the final decisions each person made, the process involved and the effort to make sense of the experience exposed the power relations between patients and physicians with respect to the biopower of gender, thereby questioning the very meanings associated with gender.

Although this work is not an ethnography, I take many cues from queer ethnography in my focus on drawing on the ways that people make sense of their experiences. This is particularly the case when those experiences challenge taken-for-granted ideas that provide stability in daily life such as gender (see Brown and Nash 2010; Rooke 2010).

Participants

I initially designed this study with a focus on gynecological care and breast cancer. As I began recruiting through internet groups, young women with BRCA diagnoses began contacting me. Although I had not initially planned to include such cases, I added them to the study because their experiences provided a useful link to those of transgender men with preventive gynecological care and cisgender women with breast cancer. Women with BRCA were engaging with preventive breast cancer care in ways similar to transgender men's engagement with gynecological care. They were also working through the same kinds of decisions as were women with breast cancer regarding mastectomies and reconstruction.

Trans Men

Thirteen transgender men participated in this research. These men were initially recruited through a snowball sample, beginning with personal contacts. I also fostered a relationship with a regional FTM support group and participated in transgender health conferences in New England. My gender nonconforming identity

Table A.1
Transgender Men

Name	Age at interview	Received care (Y/N)	Hysterectomy (Y/N)	Education	Marital and parental status[a]
Joe	36	Y	N (considering)	Bachelors	M/Y
Chris	23	Y	Y	High school	S/N
Gabe	61	Y[b]	Y	Bachelors	D/Y
Evan	60	Y	N	Bachelors	S/N
Erik	32	Y	Y	Bachelors	S/N
Kevin	26	Y	N (considering)	Masters student	S#/N
David	53	Y[b]	Y	Masters	D/Y
Jamie	27	Y	N	Masters	S#/N
Eli	33	Y	N	Bachelors	S/N
Zach	24	N	N (considering)	Bachelors	S/N
Isaac	33	Y	Y	Doctorate	S#/N
Noah	32	Y	N	Bachelors	S/N
Peter	33	Y	N	Masters	S#/N

[a] D = divorced; M = married; N = no children; S = single; S# = committed relationship; Y = has children.
[b] Indicates participant gave birth.

allowed me access to the support group and marked me as a sympathetic listener to those who agreed to participate. Upon connecting with the FTM support group, I was fully transparent about my role a researcher rather than a member.

Participants ranged in age from twenty-three to sixty-one (table A.1). All but one had experienced some kind of gynecological care, either routine screenings or treatment for a specific condition. All the men in this study had engaged in some form of medical intervention to alter their physical bodies. These interventions included any combination of hormone therapy with testosterone, top surgery (i.e., bilateral mastectomy), and bottom surgery (i.e., altering genitals via phalloplasty or metoidioplasty as well as reproductive organs via hysterectomy and/or oophorectomy). Twelve men had had top surgery, twelve were on testosterone, five had undergone hysterectomy (three were considering it), and one had scheduled a phalloplasty.

At the time of the interview, all respondents expressed a general sense of comfort with their bodies. Although some wanted to eventually alter their bodies through bilateral mastectomy or phalloplasty, given adequate financial

Table A.2
Cisgender Men

Name	Age at diagnosis	Age at interview	Education	Marital and parental status[a]
Ed	70	71	Masters	M/Y
Tim	24	28	Bachelors	S/N
Frank	55	62	Bachelors	M/Y
Ted	54	55	Masters	M/Y
James	60	61	Masters	M/Y
Larry	62	66	Bachelors	S#/N
Ezra	46	47	Doctorate	M/Y
Owen	57	66	Bachelors	M/Y
Mark	65	67	Doctorate	M/Y
Henry	53	55	Doctorate	M/Y
Mitch	51	51	Unspecified	M/Y

[a] D = divorced; M = married; N = no children; S = single; S# = committed relationship; Y = has children.

resources, all participating men had reached a point in their lives where their bodies were not discordant with their identities.

Cis Men

Eleven cisgender men agreed to share their experiences of breast cancer. Participants ranged in age from twenty-eight to seventy-one, had at least an undergraduate degree, and were white (table A.2). All but one man was married or in a committed partnership at the time of the interview. I recruited cis men at breast cancer conferences and by posting calls for participants in online forums specifically for men with breast cancer.

Cis Women

Over the course of this project, I interviewed twenty women who had breast cancer diagnoses and were treated with mastectomies (table A.3), and thirteen women who had tested positive for BRCA but did not have breast cancer (table A.4). I began recruiting participants at breast cancer conferences in New England and via personal contacts. Often, when an acquaintance learned about my dissertation topic, I would be referred to a friend who had completed treatment. The BRCA-positive women approached me when I posted calls on online venues frequented by both "previvors" (women diagnosed with BRCA) and women with breast cancer who chose mastectomies.

Table A.3
Women with BRCA

Name	Age at diagnosis	Age at interview	Reconstruction (R) or flat (F)	Education	Marital and parental status[a]	Hysterectomy or oophorectomy
Julie	30	31	R (planned)	Doctorate	S#	N
Jody	28	29	R	Bachelors	M/N	No
Alyssa	36	36	R	Masters	M/N	N
Michelle	22	28	R	Bachelors	S	No
Emily	18	22	R	Bachelors	S	No
Madison	24	28	R	Bachelors	S#	No
Julia	33	34	R	Unspecified	M/Y	No
Katie	37	45	R	Masters	M/Y	Oophorectomy
Sally	33	35	F	Masters	M/Y	Planned
Nicole	28	32	R (planned)	Unspecified	M/Y	Hysterectomy
Margaret	43	43	R	Bachelors	M/Y	Hysterectomy
Liz	29	36	F	Unspecified	M/Y	Both
Kathy	54	54	F	Masters	M/Y	Oophorectomy

[a] D = divorced; M = married; N = no children; S = single; S# = committed relationship; Y = has children.

The women in these groups are unique in the cultural story of breast cancer because they chose bilateral mastectomies, whereas other women (due to the particulars of their diagnosis) may not have had this option. Eleven of the women with BRCA had or planned to have breast reconstruction. Of the two women who live flat, one experienced severe complications after reconstruction and subsequently chose to live flat. Of the twenty women I interviewed with breast cancer, four currently have reconstructed breasts. One woman with reconstruction was considering a "deconstruction"—or removal of the implants—at the time of her interview. The remaining sixteen participants with breast cancer live flat. Of the sixteen, two women initially chose reconstructed breasts but experienced complications that led them to live flat.

Interviews

I conducted interviews in person, over the phone, or via video conferencing (Skype or FaceTime), depending on the geographical locations of the participants and their technological preferences. Interviews that were within driving distance (no more than two hours) were conducted in person whenever

Table A.4
Women with Breast Cancer

Name	Age at diagnosis	Age at interview	Reconstruction (R) or flat (F)	Education	Marital and parental status[a]
Kate	36	46	F (failed reconstruction)	Doctorate	M
Fran	52	70	F	Doctorate	M
Linda	60	63	F	Some college	S
Sandy	58	59	R	Bachelors	M
Karen	36	39	F	Doctorate	M
Edie	47	50	F	Bachelors	M
Colleen	24	34	R	Doctorate	M
Ellen[b]	38 (most recent)	56	F	Bachelors	M
Sadie	63	64	F	Masters	S/N
Ashley[b]	38, 40	41	F (separate mastectomies for primary cancers)	Unspecified	M
Samantha	45	57	F	Bachelors	M
Suzy[b]	54	54	F (one side)	Doctorate	S/N
Lorie	49	51	R (considering deconstruction)	Some college	M
Maggie	41	43	F	Doctorate	M/Y
Catherine	34	36	F	Bachelors	M
Judy[b]	45, 50	50	F	Unspecified	M
Alison	31	32	F	Doctoral student	M
Rachel	36	50	F	Some college	M
Sam	41	43	F	Masters student	M
Clare	35	39	R	Unspecified	M/Y

[a]D = divorced; M = married; N = no children; S = single; S# = committed relationship; Y = has children.

[b]Received breast cancer diagnosis twice.

possible. Skype and Facetime both provided a degree of face-to-face contact when in-person interviews were not possible. Those who chose phone interviews either did not have access to appropriate technology or they preferred the anonymity offered by a phone call. The quality of the phone interviews was not substantially different than those conducted face to face. In some cases, participants followed up our conversation by e-mailing photographs or referring me to their blogs or Facebook pages in order to illustrate the story they told.

By nature, the conversations I had with interview participants were deeply personal but very one-sided. Participants regularly asked me why I chose this research topic. I understood this question as a means for determining my trustworthiness, my knowledge about cancer, and possibly my personal perspectives on medicine. In interviews, I rarely disclosed more than a very generic explanation for why I chose this research topic, although it is, in many ways, wrapped up in my own attempts to make sense of awkward and uncomfortable medical encounters stemming from a lifetime of gender nonconformity. My ambiguity with respect to gender was a visual cue to transgender men that I was approaching their stories as more than an academic. Similarly, for women who live flat this ambiguity seemed to indicate that I could empathize with their choices.

After I provided a general explanation of the origins of the project, similar to the beginning of this appendix, participants shared their own motivations for taking part in the study. In general, they felt a need for their stories to be heard. They felt that they were on the margins of health care, and that they were largely invisible in sociocultural imaginaries of breast and gynecological care. By telling their stories, the participants could both make sense of their experiences for themselves and share this understanding with other people. Cisgender participants expressed a broad desire to make it clear to the world that there is more than one way to navigate breast cancer treatment and that breast cancer does not look the way most of us think it does. The transgender patients made it clear that gynecological care was a difficult topic, but that their stories needed to be shared with medical professionals in order for changes in care to occur.

The audience imagined by participants ranged from men (so they would become aware of their breast cancer risk), to women with breast cancer or BRCA diagnoses (so they would become aware that they have options and power in the treatment process), to physicians (so they would begin to realize how they rely on assumptions about gender, often to the detriment of their patients). The individuals who chose to participate in this research did so out of a motivation to catalyze change. Identifying similarities across experiences that seem disparate on the surface is one way to approach the community building that can eventually lead to structural change. I hope that this book takes a small step in that direction.

Appendix B

Internet Resources on Flat Closures

The following websites are a few of those now available that provide images depicting flat closures after bilateral mastectomy. Many of these websites also serve to build community among those who live flat, educate people who have recently diagnosed breast cancer and BRCA mutations about the option to live flat, and provide education and resources to health care providers about flat closures. Additionally, searching the terms "flat closure after mastectomy" or "living flat after mastectomy" will lead the reader to various articles in popular media such as the *New York Times, Huffington Post,* and other news outlets.

- Flat Friends UK. www.flatfriends.org.uk
- Flat and Fabulous. www.flatandfabulous.org
- Flat Closure Now. www.flatclosurenow.org/photo-gallery
- Not Putting on a Shirt. www.notputtingonashirt.org
- The SCAR Project by David Jay Photography. www.thescarproject.org

Acknowledgments

I began this project in earnest after leaving the urban landscape of Chicago for the low-lying mountains and fields of southern Vermont. The first person I met upon moving to a tiny village on the border of New Hampshire was the manager of the local gym. Ashley was brimming with energy when I arrived at the gym for a tour and to pick up membership information. The only mark of the breast cancer that would ultimately take her life was a brightly patterned headscarf, donned to conceal the impact of chemotherapy.

I knew Ashley for almost two years. She ran the afterschool program at the local elementary school and coached my oldest child's soccer team. She continued running (one of her many passions) even though doctors asked her to take it easy. In that first meeting I told her I was a graduate student working on my dissertation. This naturally led to a conversation about my research interests. Her eyes lit up, but she did not tell me her story. I learned it slowly, through playground conversations and chats between sets at the gym. The impact of her death lingered over that small community and reminded me daily that cancer is not just an individual's disease. It is bound up in our relationships to each other at every level.

While writing up my research, my stepfather was diagnosed with cancer. His surgeries and chemotherapy occurred as I analyzed the accounts of respondents. As difficult an experience as it was for him and our family, he and my mother reminded me that the narrative accounts that make up my data are so much more than that. Cancer touches nearly all of us. Even in communities larger than Ashley's and mine, this disease can have deep effects. Understanding and explaining the experience can be difficult. I am truly grateful to all the respondents who generously shared their stories; I hope that I have listened well.

For their patience, support, guidance, and careful engagement with my work I thank my committee of mentors: Kristen Schilt, Kate Cagney, Lauren Berlant, and Monica Casper. I am also indebted to my writing group (Abi Ocobock, Alicia Van de Vusse, Amy Brainer, and Clare Forstie) for their insightful readings of various versions of this project, and to Collin Rice, who provided valuable feedback on an early draft of this project. Bridget Nolan kept me laughing throughout the process of turning this project from a dissertation into a book and reminding me that the worst situations can be navigated if recounted with humor. I am grateful to Alison Meyers for her initial editing of this manuscript and to Kate Daniel for suggesting the title. At the time that I chose the title, I was not yet aware of Arlene Stein's book, *Unbound: Transgender Men and the Remaking of Identity.* I mean her no disrespect and hope that the similarity in our titles will be forgiven. The thoughtful engagement of Lisa Jean Moore and the anonymous reviewer truly strengthened the organization of this book. Their encouraging reviews were significant sources of motivation during the revision process. Peter Mikulas saw the potential in my work early on and has been a truly supportive advocate of this book.

Finally, I thank my family and friends: Noah, Zoe, Rowan, Nyala, and Kate; plus all of Spectrum for providing much needed comic relief and reality checks throughout this process.

Notes

Introduction

1. The Centers for Disease Control and Prevention's site for program: https://www.cdc.gov/cancer/nbccedp/.
2. I use the trans* to include those who identify as transgender, gender non-conforming, genderqueer, and the many other terms that continue to emerge in order to denote identities outside of the gender binary of man/male and woman/female.
3. The term *biocitizenship* was originally coined by Adriana Petryna (2002).
4. Although testicular examinations are a part of medical care for cisgender men, they are not effective as an early detection measure; most of these cancers are "caught" by men in everyday, non-medical situations. Prostate examination, typically comprising a blood test for prostate-specific antigens (PSA) and a manual examination, also exists but remains controversial. Neither examination is a particularly good predictor of cancer; the PSA test has a relatively high false-positive rate. In addition, the slow-growing nature of prostate cancer rarely causes death; men generally die *with* prostate cancer rather than *because* of it. As a result, treating prostate cancer remains medically controversial (Hoffman 2020).
5. Women who choose not to have reconstruction often use the term "living flat" as a more positive description of their postmastectomy choice. The term has been popularized via internet discussion boards and social media sites such as Facebook and Twitter.
6. Sociodemographic characteristics have an important correlation with the likelihood of undergoing immediate breast reconstruction, the staging of cancer at diagnosis, and the cosmetic outcomes of reconstruction (Edwards-Bennett and Brown 2011; Ballard et al. 2015; Stapleton et al. 2018). Additionally, the narratives of breast and gynecological cancers typically leave out the experiences of people of color—from involvement in clinical trials to the availability of medical images depicting the surgeries related to these cancers. While I was searching for images for chapter 3 of this book on Google, I found the repositories of medical images yielded an ubiquity of images of white women and practically no women of color or men of any race. Attention to this lack of visual representation is slowly entering popular and medical discourse (see Greaves 2018). Relevant to this study in particular is the long history of racism in the medical profession and the resultant distrust of people of color, particularly women (for a poignant example of this specific to breast cancer, see Jones 2015). My study focused on decision-making about medical interventions, so the lack of participation by people of color is unsurprising given the severe disparity in power between medical professionals and patients of color. The ability to make decisions about one's medical care requires a degree of autonomy in decision-making, which has historically been denied to patients of color.

1. Entering Enemy Territory?

1. Cancer staging is a practice used by physicians to indicate the size and extent of primary tumors, whether cancer has spread to lymph nodes, and whether there are metastases (secondary tumors). Staging helps to determine the course of treatment

as well as a patient's prognosis. Cancers can range from stage 0 (carcinoma *in situ*) to stage 5 (cancer has spread to distant tissues/organs). The higher the staging number, the more extensive the disease. Higher numbers can indicate larger tumor sizes and greater spread of the disease to other tissues beyond the primary site. In Henry's case, stage 2B is treatable. An earlier diagnosis, however, might have resulted in a less severe staging, thus improving his prognosis and requiring less extensive medical treatment.

2. A differential diagnosis is the process physicians use to differentiate between diagnoses that have similar symptoms.
3. According to the Susan G. Komen Foundation, less than 5 percent of breast cancer diagnoses occur in women under the age of forty (Komen Foundation 2020).
4. Fibroadenomas are solid tumors in the breast, and they are the most commonly found tumor in young women. These lumps tend to be surgically removed; if they are left in place, they can become cancerous. These tumors are part of a larger group of conditions called proliferative lesions without atypia, which can increase a person's risk of breast cancer. Proliferative lesions with atypia and lobular carcinoma *in situ* are two additional groups of benign conditions that can lead to increased breast cancer risk.
5. Gender capital refers to "the knowledge, resources and aspects of identity available—within a given context—that permit access to regime specific gendered identities" (Bridges 2009, 92).

2. Choosing Mastectomy

1. These scans can be time consuming and expensive. Further, not all imaging facilities are equipped with proper MRI tables for breast scans. Nor are the tests always accurate—they can miss cancers or lead to a diagnosis of cancer when it is not actually present.
2. Tissue can undergo radiation only once. If a woman has radiation therapy and her cancer returns in the same area, she cannot have radiation again, and the likelihood of having a mastectomy is high.
3. The National Cancer Institute focuses on risk up until age seventy, while the meta-analysis conducted by Chen and Parmigiani (2007) covers lifetime risk.
4. Needle biopsy is a surgical procedure done under local anesthesia. A hollow needle is inserted into suspicious tissue to remove a sample that is then examined by a pathologist.
5. Maggie used she/her pronouns during the interview.
6. David Jay's photography work in "The Scar Project" (http://www.thescarproject.org) is a notable counternarrative in which scars from breast cancer treatment are portrayed through a series of striking portraits of survivors.

3. Returning to Normal

1. The procedure is described by different names depending on the origin of the donated tissue and blood vessels. Transverse rectus abdominis myocutaneous (TRAM) flap, deep inferior epigastric perforator (DIEP) flap, and superficial inferior epigastric artery (SIEA) flap procedures all use tissue from the abdomen. The TRAM flap uses muscle and fat from the abdomen, and the DIEP flap and SIEA flap do not. The SIEA flap does not impact the muscle or fascia at all whereas the DIEP flap involves cutting through the fascia of the abdomen. Other flap procedures include the latissimus dorsi

with muscle from the upper back (often used in conjunction with silicone implants), the gluteal artery perforator (GAP) with fat from the buttocks, the transverse upper gracilis (TUG) with muscle from the upper thigh, and the profunda artery perforator (PAP) with fat from the upper thigh.

2. Medical literature suggests that although these types of physical consequences do arise from breast reconstruction, the effects are typically short term. Such impacts are expected to improve with carefully managed physical therapy, but this is not consistently included in the plan of care (Smith 2014). It stands to reason that this common lack of physical therapy could explain the experiences of women in this study.
3. One of the first images in the mainstream media of a woman living flat after breast cancer was a 1993 *New York Times Magazine* cover story depicting artist Matuschka's mastectomy scar (Ferraro 1993). The cover received a barrage of both positive and negative responses, thus opening space for ongoing efforts to bring these types of images into popular awareness.
4. These pressures are increasingly faced by men as well (see Chaline 2015; Luciano 2002).
5. The realities of publication and image rights precluded the addition of an image of a flat reconstruction here. A wide array of internet resources provide many images of flat closures and stories of those who choose to live flat. A list of some of these resources are included in appendix B.
6. This is only the case if a woman chooses reconstruction. Although surgical techniques have improved, any surgery includes the possibility of a scar. If a woman has reconstruction, the resulting breasts will overhang any scarring (however minimal) left from the mastectomy, thus making the scar extremely difficult to see.
7. I borrow this term from sociologist Kristen Barber (2016). The emotional labor that cis women participants described regarding their cis men partners and breast reconstruction was similar to the ways that women stylists explained their efforts in Barber's study of men's hair salons.
8. Breast cancer can contain proteins that respond to signals from estrogen or progesterone. These signals encourage tumor growth. Hormone therapies like tamoxifen (the most common form of hormone therapy) block those signals and prevent tumor growth, and others prohibit the production of estrogen.
9. Tamoxifen is a hormone treatment for estrogen-positive cancers. This drug blocks estrogen activity in some cells, thus helping to prevent estrogen-positive cancer cells from growing. Tamoxifen can also act like estrogen in other tissues, thus leading to potential sexual side effects for some men.
10. This same challenge to normative expectations of male sexuality is also described by trans men (see Schilt and Windsor 2014; Bishop 2016).

4. Ideologies of Gender in Surgical Cancer Care

1. Talia Mae Bettcher (2014) refers to this process of aligning gender identity with the physical body as "reality enforcement," although she is specifically discussing genitalia, not the body at large. When medical professionals engage in this reality enforcement in the treatment of individual patients, they are also contributing to enforcing the reality of binary gender and thereby shore up the biopower that gender ideologies hold.
2. The idea of body dysmorphia as a key symptom of gender dysphoria is beginning to change. In the World Professional Association for Transgender Health (WPATH) Standards of Care, medical interventions that alter the body (i.e., hormone treatments

and surgeries) are described as options, not as a prescribed course of treatment. Instead, WPATH's guidelines are explained as "flexible" and indicate that medical approaches need to be "individualized" (Coleman et al. 2012).

3. Tev spoke at length about his desire to bear children and the fact that his health care providers were shocked by his question and were never able to engage with him on this.
4. Morrow et al. (2014) also note that the rates of reconstruction are lower among racial minorities than among whites. The reasons for this remain undertheorized, and my sample was not suitable for this purpose. The intersections of race, gender, and sexuality require additional empirical consideration not only to identify patterns of disparity but also to understand how the cultural systems built around these markers of difference shape the experience of cancer and medical care more generally.

References

Abbey, Jennifer. 2012. "Breast Cancer Survivor Allowed to Swim Topless at Seattle Pool." *ABC News,* June 21. https://abcnews.go.com/US/seattle-breast-cancer-survivor-allowed-swim-topless-city/story?id=16622007.

Alderman, Amy K., Yongliang Wei, and John D. Birkmeyer. 2006. "Use of Breast Reconstruction after Mastectomy Following the Women's Health and Cancer Rights Act." *JAMA* 295 (4): 387–388.

American Board of Plastic Surgery, Inc. 2016. "About Us." https://www.abplasticsurgery.org/about-us/plastic-surgery/.

American Cancer Society. 2018. "Risk Factors for Breast Cancer in Men," April 27. http://www.cancer.org/cancer/breastcancerinmen/detailedguide/breast-cancer-in-men-risk-factors.

———. 2019. "Breast Cancer Facts & Figures 2019–2020." Atlanta: American Cancer Society. https://www.cancer.org/content/dam/cancer-org/research/cancer-facts-and-statistics/breast-cancer-facts-and-figures/breast-cancer-facts-and-figures-2019-2020.pdf.

American College of Obstetrics and Gynecology. 2006. "ACOG, AAP Develop First Collaborative Physician-focused Breastfeeding Handbook," January 25. Press release. https://web.archive.org/web/20160305202536/http://www.acog.org/About-ACOG/News-Room/News-Releases/2006/ACOG-AAP-Develop-First-Collaborative-Physician-Focused-Breastfeeding-Handbook.

———. 2011. "Health Care for Transgender Individuals." Committee Opinion. Number 512. December. https://web.archive.org/web/20191219105709/https://www.acog.org/Clinical-Guidance-and-Publications/Committee-Opinions/Committee-on-Health-Care-for-Underserved-Women/Health-Care-for-Transgender-Individuals.

———. 2012. "Ob-Gyns Recommend Women Wait 3 to 5 Years between Pap Tests." http://www.acog.org/About-ACOG/News-Room/News-Releases/2012/Ob-Gyns-Recommend-Women-Wait-3-to-5-Years-Between-Pap-Tests.

———. 2017. "ACOG Committee Opinion No. 444: Choosing the Route of Hysterectomy for Benign Disease." *Obstetrics and Gynecology* 129:e155–159.

Annandale, Ellen. (2005) 2014. "Missing Connections: Medical Sociology and Feminism." *Medical Sociology Online* 8 (2): 61–72.

———. 2009. *Women's Health and Social Change.* London: Routledge.

Annandale, Ellen, and Anne Hammerström. 2010. "Constructing the 'Gender Specific Body': A Critical Discourse Analysis of Publications in the Field of Gender-specific Medicine." *Health* 15 (6): 571–587.

Antoniou, A., P. D. P. Pharoah, S. Narod, H. A. Risch, J. E. Eyfjord, et al. 2003. "Average Risks of Breast and Ovarian Cancer Associated with BRCA1 or BRCA2 Mutations Detected in Case Series Unselected for Familial History: A Combined Analysis of 22 Studies." *American Journal of Human Genetics* 72 (5): 1117–1130.

Armstrong, Natalie. 2007. "Discourse and the Individual in Cervical Cancer Screening." *Health* 11 (1): 69–85.

Arnold, Robert M., Steven C. Martin, and Ruth M. Parker. 1988. "Taking Care of Patients: Does It Matter Whether the Physician Is a Woman?" *Western Journal of Medicine* 149 (6): 729–733.

Associated Press/Huffington Post. 2012. "Jodi Jaecks, Cancer Survivor, Allowed to Swim Topless after Fighting Seattle Pool's Ban." *Huffington Post,* June 21. https://www.huffpost.com/entry/jodi-jaecks-cancer-survivor-swimming-topless_n_1615701.

Association of American Medical Colleges. 2019a. "MD-PhD Programs by State." https://students-residents.aamc.org/applying-medical-school/article/mdphd-degree-programs-state/.

———. 2019b. "MD-PhD in 'Social Sciences or Humanities' and 'Other Non-traditional Fields of Graduate Study'—by School." https://students-residents.aamc.org/choosing-medical-career/careers-medical-research/md-phd-dual-degree-training/non-basic-science-phd-training-school/.

Atkinson, Michael. 2008. "Exploring Male Femininity in 'Crisis': Men and Cosmetic Surgery." *Body and Society* 14 (1): 67–87.

Ballard, Tiffany N. S., Yeonil Kim, Wess A. Cohen, Jennifer B. Hamill, Adeyiza O. Momoh, et al. 2015. "Sociodemographic Predictors of Breast Reconstruction Procedure Choice: Analysis of the Mastectomy Reconstruction Outcomes Consortium Study Cohort." *Plastic Surgery International.* https://doi.org/10.1155/2015/150856.

Barber, Kristen. 2016. *Styling Masculinity: Gender, Class, and Inequality in the Men's Grooming Industry.* New Brunswick, NJ: Rutgers University Press.

Bardes, Charles. 2012. "Defining 'Patient-Centered Medicine.'" *New England Journal of Medicine* 366 (9): 782–783.

Bates, Carol K., Nina Carroll, and Jennifer Potter. 2011. "The Challenging Pelvic Examination." *Journal of General Internal Medicine* 26 (6): 651–657.

Bettcher, Talia Mae. 2014. "Trapped in the Wrong Theory: Rethinking Trans Oppression and Resistance." *Signs* 39 (2): 383–406.

Bish, Alison, Amanda Ramirez, Caroline Burgess, and Myra Hunter. 2005. "Understanding Why Women Delay in Seeking Help for Breast Cancer Symptoms." *Journal of Psychosomatic Research* 58 (4): 321–326.

Bishop, Katelynn. 2016. "Body Modification and Trans Men: The Lived Realities of Gender Transition and Partner Intimacy." *Body and Society* 22 (1): 62-–91.

Bordo, Susan. 1993. *Unbearable Weight: Feminism, Western Culture, and the Body.* Berkeley: University of California Press.

———. 2009. "Twenty Years in the Twilight Zone." In *Cosmetic Surgery: A Feminist Primer,* edited by Cressida Heyes and Meredith Jones, 21–34. Surrey, United Kingdom: Ashgate.

Breastcancer.org. 2019. "U.S. Breast Cancer Statistics," June 25. https://www.breastcancer.org/symptoms/understand_bc/statistics.

Bridges, Tristan. 2009. "Gender Capital and Male Bodybuilders." *Body and Society* 15 (1): 83–107.

Bridges, Tristan, and C. J. Pascoe. 2014. "Hybrid Masculinities: New Directions in the Sociology of Men and Masculinities." *Sociology Compass* 8 (3): 246–258.

Brooke, Sebastian, John Mesa, and Mehmet Uluer. 2012. "Complications in Tissue Expander Breast Reconstruction: A Comparison of Alloderm, Demamatrix, and Flexhd Acellular Inferior Pole Dermal Slings." *Annals of Plastic Surgery* 69 (4): 347–349.

Brown, Kath, and Catherine J. Nash. 2010. "Queer Methods and Methodologies: An Introduction." In *Queer Methods and Methodologies: Intersecting Queer Theories and Social Science Research,* edited by Kath Brown and Catherine J. Nash, 1–24. Surrey, United Kingdom: Ashgate.

Butler, Judith. 2004. *Undoing Gender.* New York: Routledge.

Carpenter, Mick. 2000. "Reinforcing the Pillars: Rethinking Gender, Social Divisions, and Health." In *Gender Inequalities and Health,* edited by Ellen Annandale and Kate Hunt, 36–63. Buckingham, United Kingdom: Open University Press.

Casper, Monica J., and Laura Carpenter. 2008. "Sex, Drugs, and Politics: The HPV Vaccine for Cervical Cancer." *Sociology of Health and Illness* 30 (6): 886–899.

Centers for Disease Control and Prevention. 2019. "Leading Causes of Death—Females—All Races and Origins—United States, 2017." https://www.cdc.gov/women/lcod/2017/all-races-origins/index.htm.

Chaline, Eric. 2015. *The Temple of Perfection: A History of the Gym.* London: Reaktion Books.

Charon, Rita. 2006. *Narrative Medicine: Honoring the Stories of Illness.* Oxford: Oxford University Press.

Charon, Rita, and Martha Montello, eds. 2002. *Stories Matter: The Role of Narrative in Medical Ethics.* London: Routledge.

Charon, Rita, and Peter Wyer. 2008. "Narrative Evidence Based Medicine." *Lancet* 371 (9609): 296–297.

Chen, Sining, and Giovanni Parmigiani. 2007. "Meta-analysis of BRCA1 and BRCA2 Penetrance." *Journal of Clinical Oncology* 25 (11): 1329–1333.

Childress, Martha D. 2002. "Of Symbols and Silence: Using Narrative and Its Interpretation to Foster Physician Understanding." In *Stories Matter: The Role of Narrative in Medical Ethics,* edited by Rita Charon and Martha Montello, 119–125. London: Routledge.

Claridge, Jeffrey A., and Timothy C. Fabian. 2005. "History and Development of Evidence-Based Medicine." *World Journal of Surgery* 29 (5): 547–553.

Clarke, Juanne Nancarrow. 2004. "A Comparison of Breast, Testicular and Prostate Cancer in Mass Print Media (1996–2001). *Social Science and Medicine* 59 (3): 541–551.

Cochran, B. N., K. M. Peavy, and A. M. Cauce. 2007. "Substance Abuse Treatment Providers' Explicit and Implicit Attitudes Regarding Sexual Minorities." *Journal of Homosexuality* 53 (3): 181–207.

Coleman, Eli, Walter Bokting, Marsha Botzer, Peggy Cohen-Ketteris, Griet DeCuypere, et al., 2012. "Standards of Care for the Health of Transsexual, Transgender, and Gender Nonconforming People, Version 7." World Professional Association for Transgender Health [WPATH]. *International Journal of Transgenderism* 13 (4): 165–232. https://dx.doi.org/10.1080/15532739.2011.700873.

Connell, R. W. 1987. *Gender and Power.* Stanford, CA: Stanford University Press.

———. (1995) 2005. *Masculinities.* Cambridge: Polity Press.

Connell, Raewyn. 2012. "Gender, Health and Theory: Conceptualizing the Issue, in Local and World Perspective." *Social Science and Medicine* 74 (11): 1675–1683.

Courtenay, Will H. 2000. "Constructions of Masculinity and Their Influence on Men's Well-Being: A Theory of Gender and Health." *Social Science and Medicine* 50: 1385–1401.

Craig, Maxine Leeds. 2014. *Sorry I Don't Dance: Why Men Refuse to Move.* New York: Oxford University Press.

Crosby, Melissa A. 2010. "Reshaping You: Breast Reconstruction for Breast Cancer Patients." Houston: University of Texas M.D. Anderson Cancer Center. https://web.archive.org/web/20160418115518/https://www.mdanderson.org/patient-and-cancer-information/cancer-information/cancer-topics/cancer-treatment/surgery/breast-reconstruction/reshaping-you-booklet.pdf.

Cruz, Taylor M. 2014. “Assessing Access to Care for Transgender and Gender Nonconforming People: A Consideration of Diversity in Combating Discrimination.” *Social Science and Medicine* 110:65–73.

Cunningham, Bruce. “Discussion.” *Plastic and Reconstructive Surgery* 106 (5): 1026–1027.

Davies, Emily. 2013. “Angelina and Breast Cancer Copycat Surge: Doctor Warns Patients Are Requesting Double Mastectomies Even If They Don’t Need One.” *Daily Mail* [U.K.], October 2. http://www.dailymail.co.uk/health/article-2442141/Angelina-Jolie-copycat-surge-Double-mastectomies-unnecessary-patients-warns-doctor.html.

Davis, Georgiann. 2015. *Contesting Intersex: The Dubious Diagnosis.* New York: New York University Press.

Davis, Georgiann, Jodie M. Dewey, and Erin L. Murphy. 2016. “Giving Sex: Deconstructing Intersex and Trans Medicalization Practices.” *Gender and Society* 30 (3): 490–514.

Davis, Kate, dir. 2001. *Southern Comfort.* New York: HBO, DVD.

Davis, Kathy. 1995. *Reshaping the Female Body: The Dilemma of Cosmetic Surgery.* New York: Routledge.

———. 2003. “A ‘Dubious Equality’: Men, Women, and Cosmetic Surgery.” *Body and Society* 8 (1): 49–65.

———. 2009. “Revisiting Feminist Debates on Cosmetic Surgery: Some Reflections on Suffering, Agency, and Embodied Difference.” In *Cosmetic Surgery: A Feminist Primer,* edited by Cressida Heyes and Meredith Jones, 35–48. Surrey: Ashgate.

Dean, C., U. Chetty, and A. P. M. Forrest. 1983. “Effects of Immediate Breast Reconstruction on Psychosocial Morbidity after Mastectomy.” *Lancet* 321 (8322): 459–462.

Dole, Pamela. (1999) 2001. “Pap Smears for Survivors of Sexual Abuse.” *The Body,* May/June. https://web.archive.org/web/20181009194037/http://www.thebody.com/content/art1070. html. First published in *Positively Aware* [newsletter].

Doucleff, Michaeleen. 2013. “The Unsafe Sex: Should the World Invest More in Men’s Health?” *Shots: Health News from NPR,* May 18. http://www.npr.org/blogs/health/2013/05/17/184771915/the-unsafe-sex-should-the-world-invest-more-in-mens-health.

Dull, Diana, and Candace West. 1991. “Accounting for Cosmetic Surgery: The Accomplishment of Gender.” *Social Problems* 38 (1): 54–70.

Edwards-Bennett, Sophia M., and Carol L. Brown. 2011. “Controversies on Cosmetic Outcomes in Black Women after Breast Conservation Therapy: Hyperperception or Hyperpigmentation?” *Clinical, Cosmetic, and Investigational Dermatology* 4:15–17.

Elmore, Joann G., Gary M. Longton, Patricia A. Carney, Berta M. Geller, Tracy Onega, et al. 2015. “Diagnostic Concordance among Pathologists Interpreting Breast Biopsy Specimens.” *JAMA* 313 (11): 1122–1132.

Elson, Jean. 2004. *Am I Still a Woman: Hysterectomy and Gender Identity.* Philadelphia: Temple University Press.

Epner, Daniel E., and Walter F. Baile. 2012. “Patient-Centered Care: The Key to Cultural Differences.” *Annals of Oncology* 3:33–42.

Epstein, Steven. 2007. *Inclusion: The Politics of Difference in Medical Research.* Chicago: University of Chicago Press.

Ericksen, Julia A. 2008. *Taking Charge of Breast Cancer.* Berkeley: University of California Press.

Eyler, A. Evan. 2007. “Primary Medical Care of the Gender Variant Patient.” In *Principles of Transgender Medicine and Surgery,* edited by Randi Ettner, Stan Monstrey, and A. Evan Eyler, 15–32. New York: Haworth Press.

Fassin, Didier. 2009. "Another Politics of Life Is Possible." *Theory, Culture, and Society* 26 (5): 44–60.

Fausto-Sterling, Anne. 1993. "The Five Sexes: Why Male and Female Are Not Enough." *The Sciences,* March/April: 20–25.

———. 2000. *Sexing the Body: Gender, Politics, and the Construction of Sexuality.* New York: Basic Books.

Felski, Rita. 2006. "'Because It Is Beautiful:' New Feminist Perspectives on Beauty." *Feminist Theory* 7 (2): 273–282.

Ferraro, Susan. 1993. "The Anguished Politics of Breast Cancer." *New York Times Magazine,* August 15, p. 25. http://www.beautyoutofdamage.com/nytimesaug151993.pdf.

Ferro, Shaunacy. 2013. "A Guide to Not Saying Dumb Things about Angelina Jolie's Double Mastectomy." *Popular Science,* May 16. http://www.popsci.com/science/article/2013-05/breaking-down-angelina-jolies-breast-cancer-bombshell.

Foucault, Michel. 1978. *The History of Sexuality,* Vol. 1: *An Introduction.* New York: Vintage Books.

———. 1988. *Technologies of the Self: A Seminar with Michel Foucault.* Edited by Luther H. Martin, Huck Gutman, and Patrick H. Hutton. Amherst: University of Massachusetts Press.

Frank, Arthur W. 1995. *The Wounded Storyteller: Body, Illness, and Ethics.* Chicago: University of Chicago Press.

———. 2000. "Illness and Autobiographical Work: Dialogue as Narrative Destabilization." *Qualitative Sociology* 23 (1): 135–156.

Friedman, Asia. 2013. *Blind to Sameness: Sexpectations and the Social Construction of Male and Female Bodies.* Chicago: University of Chicago Press.

Frost, Marlene H., Daniel J. Schaid, Thomas A. Sellers, Jeffrey M. Slezak, Phillip G. Arnold, et al. 2000. "Long-Term Satisfaction and Psychological and Social Function Following a Bilateral Prophylactic Mastectomy." *JAMA* 284 (3): 319–324.

Furnham, A., and Swami, V. 2007. "Perceptions of Female Buttocks and Breast Size in Profile." *Social Behavior and Personality* 35 (1): 1–8.

Gagné, Patricia, and Deanna McGaughey. 2002. "Designing Women: Cultural Hegemony and the Exercise of Power among Women Who Have Undergone Elective Mammoplasty." *Gender and Society* 16 (6): 814–838.

Gillespie, Rosemary. 2002. "Architecture and Power: A Family Planning Clinic as a Case Study." *Health and Place* 8 (3): 211–220.

Gimlin, Debra. 2002. *Body Work: Beauty and Self-Image in American Culture.* Berkeley: University of California Press.

———. 2007. "What Is Body Work?" *Sociology Compass* 1 (1): 353–370.

———. 2010. "The Other of Aesthetic Plastic Surgery." *Body and Society* 16 (4): 57–76.

———. 2013. "'Too Good to Be Real': The Obviously Augmented Breast in Women's Narratives of Cosmetic Surgery." *Gender and Society* 27 (6): 913–934.

Grant, Jamie M., Lisa A. Mottet, Justin Tanis, Jack Harrison, Jody L. Herman, and Mara Keisling. 2011. *Injustice at Every Turn: A Report of the National Transgender Discrimination Survey.* Washington, DC: National Center for Transgender Equality.

Greaves, Kayla. 2018. "Black Women Are Underrepresented in the Breast Cancer Community, Even though They're More Likely to Die from the Disease." *Bustle,* October 23. https://www.bustle.com/p/black-women-are-underrepresented-in-the-breast-cancer-community-even-though-theyre-more-likely-to-die-from-the-disease-12232237.

Grimmer, Laura, Erik Liederbach, Jose Velasco, Catherine Pesce, Chi-Hsiung Wan, and Katharine Yao. 2015. "Variation in Contralateral Prophylactic Mastectomy Rates

According to Racial Groups in Young Women with Breast Cancer, 1998–2011: A Report from the National Cancer Data Base." *Journal of the American College of Surgeons* 221 (1): 187–196.

Gross, Terry. 2015. "Surgeon Seeks to Help Women Navigate Breast Cancer Treatment." Interview with Dr. Elisa Port. *Shots: Health News from NPR,* September 22. http://www.npr.org/sections/health-shots/2015/09/22/442343578/surgeon-seeks-to-help-women-navigate-breast-cancer-treatment.

Gurevich, Maria, Scott Bishop, Jo Bower, Monika Malka, and Joyce Nyhof-Young. 2004. "(Dis)embodying Gender and Sexuality in Testicular Cancer." *Social Science and Medicine* 58:1597–1607.

Hagen, D. Brienne, and M. Paz Galupo. 2014. "Trans* Individuals' Experiences of Gendered Language with Health Care Providers: Recommendations for Practitioners." *International Journal of Transgenderism* 15:16–34.

Hallowell, Nina, and Julia Lawton. 2002. "Negotiating Present and Future Selves: Managing the Risk of Hereditary Ovarian Cancer by Prophylactic Surgery." *Health* 6 (4): 423–443.

Hamblin, James. 2016. "Evidence of the Superiority of Female Doctors." *Atlantic,* December 19. https://www.theatlantic.com/health/archive/2016/12/female-doctors-superiority/511034/.

Hammarström, Anne, Klara Johansson, Ellen Annandale, Christina Ahlgren, Lena Aléx, et al. 2014. "Central Gender Theoretical Concepts in Health Research: The State of the Art." *Journal of Epidemiology and Community Health* 68:185–190.

Harding, Sandra. 2004a. "Rethinking Standpoint Epistemology: What Is 'Strong Objectivity'?" In *Feminist Perspectives on Social Research,* edited by Sharlene Nagy Hesse-Biber and Michelle L. Yaiser, 39–64. New York: Oxford University Press.

———. 2004b. "A Socially Relevant Philosophy of Science? Resources from Standpoint Theory's Controversiality." *Hypatia* 19 (1): 25–47.

Hart, Chloe Grace, Aliya Saperstein, Devon Magliozzi, and Laurel Westbrook. 2019. "Gender and Health: Beyond Binary Categorical Measurement." *Journal of Health and Social Behavior* 60 (1): 101–118.

Hawley, Sarah T., Reshma Jagsi, and Monica Marrow. 2014. "Social and Clinical Determinants of Contralateral Prophylactic Mastectomy." *JAMA Surgery* 149 (6): 582–589.

Hesse-Biber, Sharlene. 2014. *Waiting for Cancer to Come: Women's Experiences with Genetic Testing and Medical Decision Making for Breast and Ovarian Cancer.* Ann Arbor: University of Michigan Press.

Heyes, Cressida, and Meredith Jones. 2009. "Cosmetic Surgery in the Age of Gender." In *Cosmetic Surgery: A Feminist Primer,* edited by Cressida Heyes and Meredith Jones, 1–17. Surrey, United Kingdom: Ashgate.

Hoffman, Richard M. 2020. "Screening for Prostate Cancer." *UpToDate,* March 20. http://www.uptodate.com/contents/screening-for-prostate-cancer.

Hollander, Jocelyn A. 2001. "Vulnerability and Dangerousness: The Construction of Gender through Conversation about Violence." *Gender and Society* 15 (1): 83–109.

Howlader, N., A. M. Noone, M. Krapcho, D. Miller, A. Brest, et al., eds. 2019. *SEER Cancer Statistics Review, 1975–2016.* Bethesda, MD: National Cancer Institute. https://seer.cancer.gov/csr/1975_2016/.

Institute of Medicine. 2011. *The Health of Lesbian, Gay, Bisexual, and Transgender People: Building a Foundation for a Better Understanding.* Washington, DC: National Academies Press.

Jagsi, Reshma, Jing Jiang, Adeyiza O. Momoh, Amy Alderman, Sharon H. Giordano, et al. 2014. "Trends and Variation in Use of Breast Reconstruction in Patients with Breast Cancer Undergoing Mastectomy in the United States." *Journal of Clinical Oncology* 32 (9): 919–930.

Jain, S. Lochlann. 2013. *Malignant: How Cancer Becomes Us.* Berkeley: University of California Press.

James, S. E, J. L. Herman, S. Rankin, M. Keisling, L. Mottet, and M. Anafi. 2016. *The Report of the 2015 U.S. Transgender Survey.* Washington D.C.: National Center for Transgender Equality.

Jin, Jill. 2013. "Women with Breast Cancer Who Opt for Contralateral Prophylactic Mastectomy Might Overestimate Risk." *JAMA* 310 (15): 1548.

Johnson, Austin H. 2015. "Normative Accountability: How the Medical Model Influences Transgender Identities and Experiences." *Sociology Compass* 99:803–813.

Jolie, Angelina. 2013. "My Medical Choice." *New York Times,* May 14. http://www.nytimes.com/2013/05/14/opinion/my-medical-choice.html.

Jones, Diana. 2015. "Knowledge, Beliefs, and Feelings about Breast Cancer: The Perspective of African American Women." *Association of Black Nursing Faculty Journal* 26 (1): 5–10.

Katz, Steven J., and Monica Morrow. 2013. "Contralateral Prophylactic Mastectomy for Breast Cancer: Addressing Peace of Mind." *JAMA* 310 (8): 793–794.

Kerlikowske, Karla, Weiwei Zhu, Rebecca A. Hubbard, Berta Geller, Kim Dittus, et al. 2013. "Outcomes of Screening Mammography by Frequency, Breast Density, and Postmenopausal Hormone Therapy." *JAMA Internal Medicine* 173 (9): 807–816.

Kessler, Suzanne J., and Wendy McKenna. (1978) 1985. *Gender: An Ethnomethodological Approach.* Chicago: University of Chicago Press. First published by Wiley Interscience (New York).

King, M. C., J. H. Marks, J. B. Mandell, and New York Breast Cancer Study Group. 2003. "Breast and Ovarian Cancer Risks due to Inherited Mutations in BRCA1 and BRCA2." *Science* 302 (5645): 643–646.

King, Samantha. 2006. *Pink Ribbons, Inc.: Breast Cancer and the Politics of Philanthropy.* Minneapolis: University of Minnesota Press.

Klawiter, Maren. 2008. *The Biopolitics of Breast Cancer: Changing Cultures of Disease and Activism.* Minneapolis: University of Minnesota Press.

Komen Foundation. 2020. "Breast Cancer Statistics." *Susan G. Komen,* May 18. http://ww5.komen.org/BreastCancer/Statistics.html.

Lefebvre, Guylaine, Catherine Allaire, John Jeffrey, George Vilos, Jagmit Arneja, et al., and the Clinical Practice Gynaecology Committee and Executive Committeee and Council, Society of Obstetricians and Gynaecologists of Canada. 2002. "SOGC Clinical Guidelines. Hysterectomy." *Journal of Obstetrics and Gynaecology Canada* 24 (1): 37–61.

Legato, Marianne J. 2004. "Gender-Specific Medicine: The View from Salzburg." *Gender and Medicine* 1 (2): 61–63.

Lewin, Ellen, and Virginia Olesen, eds. 1985. *Women, Health, and Healing.* London: Tavistock.

Loe, Meika. 2004. *The Rise of Viagra: How the Little Blue Pill Changed Sex in America.* New York: New York University Press.

———. 2006. "The Viagra Blues: Embracing and Resisting the Viagra Body." In *Medicalized Masculinities,* edited by Dana Rosenfeld and Christopher A. Faircloth, 21–44. Philadelphia: Temple University Press.

Longino, Helen. 1990. *Science as Social Knowledge: Values and Objectivity in Scientific Inquiry.* Princeton, NJ: Princeton University Press.

Lucal, Betsy. 2008. "Building Boxes and Policing Boundaries: (De)Constructing Intersexuality, Transgender, and Bisexuality." *Sociology Compass* 2 (2): 519–536.

Luciano, Lynne. 2002. *Looking Good: Male Body Image in Modern America.* New York: Hill and Wang.

Lurie, S. 2005. Identifying Training Needs of Health-Care Providers Related to Treatment and Care of Transgendered Patients: A Qualitative Needs Assessment Conducted in New England. *International Journal of Transgenderism* 8 (2–3): 93–112.

Mazure, Carolyn, and Daniel P. Jones. 2015. "Twenty Years and Still Counting Including Women as Participants and Studying Sex and Gender in Biomedical Research." *BMC Women's Health* 15:94.

Metzl, Jonathan, and Anna Kirkland, eds. 2010. *Against Health: How Health Became the New Morality.* New York: New York University Press.

Meyerowitz, Joanne. 2002. *How Sex Changed: A History of Transsexuality in the United States.* Cambridge, MA: Harvard University Press.

Moore, Sarah E. H. 2010. "Is the Healthy Body Gendered? Toward A Feminist Critique of the New Paradigm of Health." *Body and Society* 16:95–118.

Morgan, Kathryn Pauly. 1991. "Women and the Knife: Cosmetic Surgery and the Colonization of Women's Bodies." *Hypatia* 6 (3): 25–53.

Morgen, Sandra. 2002. *Into Our Own Hands: The Women's Health Movement in the United States, 1969–1990.* New Brunswick, NJ: Rutgers University Press.

Morrow, Monica, Yun Li, Amy K. Alderman, Reshma Jagsi, Ann S. Hamilton, et al. 2014. "Access to Breast Reconstruction after Mastectomy: Patient Perspectives on Reconstruction Decision Making." *JAMA Surgery* 149 (10): 1015–1021.

Mukherjee, Siddhartha. 2010. *The Emperor of All Maladies: A Biography of Cancer.* New York: Scribner.

Nahabedian, Maurice. 2020. "Overview of Breast Reconstruction." *UpToDate,* April 14. http://www.uptodate.com/contents/overview-of-breast-reconstruction.

National Cancer Institute. 2018. "BRCA Mutations: Cancer Risk and Genetic Testing." http://www.cancer.gov/cancertopics/factsheet/Risk/BRCA.

Negrin, Llewellyn. 2002. "Cosmetic Surgery and the Eclipse of Identity." *Body and Society* 8 (4): 21–42.

Nordmarken, Sonny, and Reese Kelly. 2014. "Limiting Transgender Health: Administrative Violence and Microaggressions in Health Care Systems." In *Health Care Disparities and the LGBT Population,* edited by Vickie L. Harvey and Teresa Heinz Housel, 143–166. Plymouth: Lexington Books.

Norman, Moss E. 2011. "Embodying the Double-Bind of Masculinity: Young Men and Discourses of Normalcy, Health, Heterosexuality, and Individualism." *Men and Masculinities* 14 (4): 430–449.

Oeffinger, Kevin, Elizabeth T. H. Fontham, Ruth Etzioni, Abbe Herzig, James S. Michaelson, et al. 2015. "Breast Cancer Screening for Women at Average Risk: 2015 Guideline Update from the American Cancer Society." *JAMA* 314 (15): 1599–1614.

Oliffe, John. 2009. "Health Behaviours, Prostate Cancer, and Masculinities: A Life Course Perspective." *Men and Masculinities* 11 (3): 346–366.

Ong, Aihwa. 2011. "Translating Gender Justice in Southeast Asia: Situated Ethics, NGOs, and Bio-Welfare." *Journal of Women of the Middle East and the Islamic World* 9:26–48.

Osman, Fahima, Fady Saleh, Timothy D. Jackson, Mark A. Corrigan, and Tulin Cil. 2013. "Increased Postoperative Complications in Bilateral Mastectomy Patients Compared to

Unilateral Mastectomy: An Analysis of the NSQIP Database." *Annals of Surgical Oncology* 20 (10): 3212–3127.

Parker, Patricia A. 2004. "Breast Reconstruction and Psychosocial Adjustment: What Have We Learned and Where Do We Go from Here?" *Seminars in Plastic Surgery* 18 (2): 131–138.

Parks, Anna L., and Rita F. Redberg. 2017. "Women in Medicine and Patient Outcomes: Equal Rights for Better Work?" *JAMA Internal Medicine* 177 (2): 161.

Pemmaraju, N., M. F. Munsell, G. N. Hortobagyi, and S. H. Giordano. 2012. "Retrospective Review of Male Breast Cancer Patients: Analysis of Tamoxifen-Related Side-Effects." *Annals of Oncology* 23 (6): 1471–1474.

Petryna, Adriana. 2002. *Life Exposed: Biological Citizens after Chernobyl.* Princeton, NJ: Princeton University Press.

Pinkhasov, R. M., J. Wong, J. Kashanian, M. Lee, D. B. Samadi, et al. 2010. "Are Men Shortchanged on Health? Perspectives on Health Care Utilization and Health Risk Behavior in Men and Women in the United States." *International Journal of Clinical Practice* 64 (4): 475–487.

Potts, Laura K. 2000. "Publishing the Personal: Autobiographical Narratives of Breast Cancer and the Self." In *Ideologies of Breast Cancer,* edited by Laura K. Potts, 98–130. New York: St. Martin's Press.

Preves, Sharon E. 2000. "Negotiating the Constraints of Gender Binarism: Intersexuals' Challenge to Gender Categorization." *Current Sociology* 48 (3): 27–50.

———. 2002. "Sexing the Intersexed: An Analysis of Sociocultural Responses to Intersexuality." *Signs* 27(2): 523–556.

Prosser, Jay. 1998. *Second Skins: The Body Narratives of Transsexuality.* New York: Columbia University Press.

Rabinowitz, Barbara. 2013. "Psychological Aspects of Breast Reconstruction." In *Oncoplastic and Reconstructive Breast Surgery,* edited by Cicero Urban and Mario Rietjens, 423–429. Milan: Springer-Verlag Italia.

Read, Jen'nan Ghazal, and Bridget K. Gorman. 2010. "Gender and Health Inequality." *Annual Review of Sociology* 36:317–386.

Reilly, Rick. 2019. "Swimming Upstream." *ESPN,* June 26. https://www.espn.com/espn/story/_/id/8098241/swimming-breast-removal.

Repo, Jemima. 2013. "The Biopolitical Birth of Gender: Social Control, Hermaphroditism, and the New Sexual Apparatus." *Alternatives: Global, Local, Political* 38 (3): 228–244.

———. 2016. *The Biopolitics of Gender.* Oxford: Oxford University Press.

Risberg, Gunilla, Eva E. Johansson, Göran Westman, and Katarina Hamberg. 2003. "Gender in Medicine—An Issue for Women Only? A Survey of Physician Teachers' Gender Attitudes." *International Journal for Equity in Health* 2:10.

Rollston, Rebekah. 2019. "Promoting Cervical Cancer Screening among Female-to-Male Transmasculine Patients." Policy Brief. Boston: Fenway Institute.

Rooke, Alison. 2010. "Queer in the Field: On Emotions, Temporality, and Performativity in Ethnography." In *Queer Methods and Methodologies: Intersecting Queer Theories and Social Science Research,* edited by Kath Brown and Catherine J. Nash, 24–40. Surrey, United Kingdom: Ashgate.

Rose, Nikolas. 2007. *The Politics of Life Itself: Biomedicine, Power, and Subjectivity in the Twenty-First Century.* Princeton, NJ: Princeton University Press.

Rose, Nikolas, and Carlos Novas. 2005. "Biological Citizenship." In *Global Assemblages: Technology, Politics, and Ethics as Anthropological Problems,* edited by Aihwa Ong and Stephen Collier, 439–463. Oxford: Blackwell.

Rosenberg, Shoshana M., and Ann H. Partridge. 2014. "Contralateral Prophylactic Mastectomy: An Opportunity for Shared Decision Making." *JAMA Surgery* 149 (6): 589–590.

Rosenfeld, Dana, and Christopher A. Faircloth. 2006. "Medicalized Masculinities: The Missing Link?" In *Medicalized Masculinities,* edited by Dana Rosenfeld and Christopher A. Faircloth, 1–20. Philadelphia: Temple University Press.

Rowland, Julia H., Joe Dioso, Jimmie C. Holland, Ted Chaglassian, and David Kinne. 2000. "Breast Reconstruction after Mastectomy: Who Seeks It, Who Refuses? *Plastic and Reconstructive Surgery* 95 (5): 812–822.

Rubin, Henry. 2003. *Self-Made Men: Identity and Embodiment among Transsexual Men.* Nashville: Vanderbilt University Press.

Ruzek, Sheryl Burt. 1978. *The Women's Health Movement: Feminist Alternatives to Medical Control.* New York: Praeger.

Saha, Somanth, Mary Catherine Beach, and Lisa A. Cooper. 2008. "Patient Centeredness, Cultural Competence and Healthcare Quality." *Journal of the National Medical Association* 100 (11): 1275–1285.

Schilt, Kristen. 2010. *Just One of the Guys: Transgender Men and the Persistence of Gender Inequality.* Chicago: University of Chicago Press.

Schilt, Kristen, and Laurel Westbrook. 2009. "Doing Gender, Doing Heteronormativity: 'Gender Normals,' Transgender People, and the Social Maintenance of Heterosexuality." *Gender and Society* 23 (4): 440–464.

Schilt, Kristen, and Elroi Windsor. 2014. "The Sexual Habitus of Transgender Men: Negotiating Sexuality through Gender." *Journal of Homosexuality* 16 (5): 732–748.

Schippers, Mimi. 2007. "Recovering the Feminine Other: Masculinity, Femininity, and Gender Hegemony." *Theory and Society* 36:85–102.

Schumann, John Henning, and Sarah-Anne Henning Schumann. 2016. "Patients Cared for by Female Doctors Fare Better Than Those Treated by Men." *Shots: Health News from NPR,* December 19. https://www.npr.org/sections/health-shots/2016/12/19/506144346/patients-cared-for-by-female-doctors-fare-better-than-those-treated-by-men.

Schwartz, Pepper. 2007. "The Social Construction of Heterosexuality." In *The Sexual Self: The Construction of Sexual Scripts,* edited by Michael Kimmel, 80–92. Nashville: Vanderbilt University Press.

Seymore, Carolyn, Robert H. DuRant, Susan Jay, David Freeman, Lily Gomez, et al. 1986. "Influence of Position during Examination, and Sex of Examiner on Patient Anxiety during Pelvic Examination." *Journal of Pediatrics* 108 (2): 312–317.

Shildrick, Margrit. 2010. "Some Reflections on the Socio-cultural and Bioscientific Limits of Bodily Integrity." *Body and Society* 16 (3): 11–22.

Sledge, Piper. 2019. "From Decision to Incision: Ideologies of Gender in Surgical Cancer Care." *Social Science and Medicine* 239:112550.

Smith, Susan L. 2014. "Functional Morbidity Following Latissimus Dorsi Flap Breast Reconstruction." *Journal of the Advanced Practitioner in Oncology* 5 (3): 181–187.

Spade, Dean. 2003. "Resisting Medicine, Re/Modeling Gender." *Berkeley Women's Law Journal* 18 (1): 15–37.

———. 2011. "About Purportedly Gendered Body Parts." DeanSpade.net. http://www.deanspade.net/wp-content/uploads/2011/02/Purportedly-Gendered-Body-Parts.pdf.

Speirs, Valerie, Steven Pollock, Abeer M. Shaaban, and Andrew M. Hanby. 2010. "Problems (and Solutions) in the Study of Male Breast Cancer." *Rare Tumors* 2 (2): e28.

Speirs, Valerie, and Abeer M. Shaaban. 2009. "The Rising Incidence of Male Breast Cancer." *Breast Cancer Research and Treatment.* 115:429–430.

Springer, Kristen W., Olena Hankivsky, and Lisa M. Bates. 2012. "Gender and Health: Relational, Intersectional, and Biosocial Approaches." *Social Science and Medicine* 74:1661–1666.

Stapleton, Sahael M., Tawakalitu O. Oseni, Yanik J. Bababekov, Ya-Ching Hung, and David Chang. 2018. "Breast Cancer Diagnosis in the United States." *JAMA Surgery* 153 (6): 594–595.

Stavrou, Demetris, Oren Weissman, Anna Polyniki, Neofytos Papageoriou, Joseph Haik, et al. 2009. "Quality of Life after Breast Cancer Surgery with or without Reconstruction." *Eplasty* 9:e18.

Stibbe, Arran. 2004. "Health and Social Construction of Masculinity in Men's Health Magazine." *Men and Masculinities* 7 (1): 31–51.

Stuart, Avelie, and Ngaire Donaghue. 2011. "Choosing to Conform: The Discursive Complexities of Choice in Relation to Feminine Beauty Practices." *Feminism and Psychology* 22 (1): 98–121.

Sulik, Gayle. 2011. *Pink Ribbon Blues: How Breast Cancer Culture Undermines Women's Health.* New York: Oxford University Press.

Sullivan, Nikki. 2008. "The Role of Medicine in the (Trans)Formation of 'Wrong' Bodies." *Body and Society* 14 (1): 105–116.

Sullivan, Stephen R., Derek R. D. Fletcher, Casey D. Isom, and Frank F. Isik. 2008. "True Incidence of All Complications Following Immediate and Delayed Breast Reconstruction." *Plastic and Reconstructive Surgery* 122 (1): 19–28.

Sur, Roger L., and Phillip Dahm. 2011. "History of Evidence-Based Medicine." *Indian Journal of Urology* 27 (4): 487–489.

Temkin, Sarah M., and Kimberly Kho. 2014. "Hysterectomy." U.S. Office of Women's Health. http://womenshealth.gov/publications/our-publications/fact-sheet/hysterectomy.html.

Tracy, Michaela S., Shoshana Rosenberg, Laura Dominici, and Ann H. Partridge. 2013. "Contralateral Prophylactic Mastectomy in Women with Breast Cancer: Trends, Predictors, and Areas for Future Research." *Breast Cancer Research and Treatment* 140 (3): 447–452.

Tsugawa, Yusuke, Anupam B. Jena, Jose F. Figueroa, E. John Orav, Daniel M. Blumenthal, and Ashish K. Jha. 2017. "Physician Gender and Outcomes of Hospitalized Medicare Beneficiaries in the U.S." *JAMA Internal Medicine* 177 (2): 206–213.

Tuttle, Todd M., Elizabeth B. Habermann, Erin H. Grund, Todd J. Morris, and Beth A. Virnig. 2007. "Increasing Use of Contralateral Prophylactic Mastectomy for Breast Cancer Patients: A Trend toward More Aggressive Treatment." *Journal of Clinical Oncology* 25 (33): 5203–5209.

Underman, Kelly. 2015. "Playing Doctor: Simulation in Medical School as Affective Practice." *Social Science and Medicine* 136–137:180–188.

Vaidya, V., G. Partha, and M. Karmakar. 2012. "Gender Differences in Utilization of Preventive Care Services in the United States." *Journal of Women's Health* 21 (2): 140–145.

Valdes, Manuel. 2012. "Seattle Pool Allows Topless Breast Cancer Survivor." *Washington Times,* June 21. https://www.washingtontimes.com/news/2012/jun/21/seattle-pool-allows-topless-breast-cancer-survivor/.

Van Trotsenberg, Michael A. A. 2009. "Gynecological Aspects of Transgender Healthcare." *International Journal of Transgenderism* 11:238–246.

Vaughan, Alexa. 2012. "After Months of Trying, a Seattle Woman Who Underwent a Double Mastectomy Has Won Permission to Swim Topless in City Pools." *Seattle Times,*

June 20. https://www.seattletimes.com/seattle-news/breast-cancer-survivor-fights-city-wins-right-to-swim-in-pool-topless/.

Wallace, Kelly. 2014. "Why Are We Still So Squeamish about Breastfeeding?" CNN, August 29. http://www.cnn.com/2014/08/29/living/breastfeeding-attitudes-parents/.

Watson, Jonathan. 2000. *Male Bodies: Health, Culture, and Identity.* Philadelphia: Open University Press.

West, Candace, and Don Zimmerman. 1987. "Doing Gender." *Gender and Society* 1 (2): 125–151.

———. 2009. "Accounting for Doing Gender." *Gender and Society* 23 (1): 112–122.

Westbrook, Laurel. 2008. "Vulnerable Subjecthood: The Risks and Benefits of the Struggle for Hate Crime Legislation." *Berkeley Journal of Sociology* 52:3–24.

Westbrook, Laurel, and Kristen Schilt. 2014. "Doing Gender, Determining Gender: Transgender People, Gender Panics, and the Maintenance of the Sex/Gender/Sexuality System." *Gender and Society* 28 (1): 32–57.

Wienke, Chris. 2000. "Better Loving through Chemistry: How New Impotence Treatment Technologies Promise to Change Male Sexuality." *Disclosure* 9:69–93.

———. 2005. "Male Sexuality, Medicalization, and the Marketing of Cialis and Levitra." *Sexuality and Culture* 9 (4): 29–57.

———. 2006. "Sex the Natural Way: The Marketing of Cialis and Levitra." In *Medicalized Masculinities,* edited by Dana Rosenfeld and Christopher A. Faircloth, 45–64. Philadelphia: Temple University Press.

Wilkins, Edwin G., Paul S. Cederna, Julie C. Lower, Jennifer A. Davis, Hyungjin Myra Kim, et al. 2000. "Prospective Analysis of Psychosocial Outcomes in Breast Reconstruction: One-Year Postoperative Results from the Michigan Breast Reconstruction Outcome Study." *Plastic and Reconstructive Surgery* 106 (5):1014–1025.

Williams, Allison. 2002. "Changing Geographies of Care: Employing the Concept of Therapeutic Landscapes as a Framework in Examining Home Space." *Social Science and Medicine* 55 (1):141–154.

Williams, Gareth. 1984. "The Genesis of Chronic Illness: Narrative Reconstruction." *Sociology of Health and Illness* 6:175–200.

Young, Iris Marion. 1980. "Throwing Like a Girl: A Phenomenology of Feminine Body Comportment Motility and Spatiality." *Human Studies* 3 (2): 137–156.

———. 2005. *On Female Body Experience: "Throwing Like a Girl" and Other Essays.* New York: Oxford University Press.

Young, Kathryne M. 2017. "Masculine Compensation and Masculine Balance: Notes on the Hawaiian Cockfight." *Social Forces* 95 (4): 1341–1370.

Zeichner, S. B., S. B. Zeichner, A. L. Ruiz, N. J. Markward, and E. Rodriguez. 2014. "Improved Long-Term Survival with Contralateral Prophylactic Mastectomy among Young Women." *Asian Pacific Journal of Cancer Prevention* 15 (3): 1155–1162.

Index

Note: Pages in *italic type* refer to illustrative matter.

About the Author

Piper Sledge is an assistant professor of sociology and director of the Gender and Sexuality Studies Program at Bryn Mawr College in Pennsylvania.

Available titles in the Critical Issues in Health and Medicine series:

Emily K. Abel, *Prelude to Hospice: Florence Wald, Dying People, and Their Families*
Emily K. Abel, *Suffering in the Land of Sunshine: A Los Angeles Illness Narrative*
Emily K. Abel, *Tuberculosis and the Politics of Exclusion: A History of Public Health and Migration to Los Angeles*
Marilyn Aguirre-Molina, Luisa N. Borrell, and William Vega, eds., *Health Issues in Latino Males: A Social and Structural Approach*
Anne-Emanuelle Birn and Theodore M. Brown, eds., *Comrades in Health: U.S. Health Internationalists, Abroad and at Home*
Karen Buhler-Wilkerson, *False Dawn: The Rise and Decline of Public Health Nursing*
Susan M. Chambré, *Fighting for Our Lives: New York's AIDS Community and the Politics of Disease*
James Colgrove, Gerald Markowitz, and David Rosner, eds., *The Contested Boundaries of American Public Health*
Cynthia A. Connolly, *Children and Drug Safety: Balancing Risk and Protection in Twentieth-Century America*
Cynthia A. Connolly, *Saving Sickly Children: The Tuberculosis Preventorium in American Life, 1909–1970*
Brittany Cowgill, *Rest Uneasy: Sudden Infant Death Syndrome in Twentieth-Century America*
Patricia D'Antonio, *Nursing with a Message: Public Health Demonstration Projects in New York City*
Tasha N. Dubriwny, *The Vulnerable Empowered Woman: Feminism, Postfeminism, and Women's Health*
Edward J. Eckenfels, *Doctors Serving People: Restoring Humanism to Medicine through Student Community Service*
Julie Fairman, *Making Room in the Clinic: Nurse Practitioners and the Evolution of Modern Health Care*
Jill A. Fisher, *Medical Research for Hire: The Political Economy of Pharmaceutical Clinical Trials*
Charlene Galarneau, *Communities of Health Care Justice*
Alyshia Gálvez, *Patient Citizens, Immigrant Mothers: Mexican Women, Public Prenatal Care, and the Birth-weight Paradox*
Janet Greenlees, *When the Air Became Important: A Social History of the New England and Lancashire Textile Industries*
Gerald N. Grob and Howard H. Goldman, *The Dilemma of Federal Mental Health Policy: Radical Reform or Incremental Change?*
Gerald N. Grob and Allan V. Horwitz, *Diagnosis, Therapy, and Evidence: Conundrums in Modern American Medicine*
Rachel Grob, *Testing Baby: The Transformation of Newborn Screening, Parenting, and Policymaking*
Mark A. Hall and Sara Rosenbaum, eds., *The Health Care "Safety Net" in a Post-Reform World*
Laura L. Heinemann, *Transplanting Care: Shifting Commitments in Health and Care in the United States*
Laura D. Hirshbein, *American Melancholy: Constructions of Depression in the Twentieth Century*
Laura D. Hirshbein, *Smoking Privileges: Psychiatry, the Mentally Ill, and the Tobacco Industry in America*

Timothy Hoff, *Practice under Pressure: Primary Care Physicians and Their Medicine in the Twenty-first Century*

Beatrix Hoffman, Nancy Tomes, Rachel N. Grob, and Mark Schlesinger, eds., *Patients as Policy Actors*

Ruth Horowitz, *Deciding the Public Interest: Medical Licensing and Discipline*

Powel Kazanjian, *Frederick Novy and the Development of Bacteriology in American Medicine*

Claas Kirchhelle, *Pyrrhic Progress: The History of Antibiotics in Anglo-American Food Production*

Rebecca M. Kluchin, *Fit to Be Tied: Sterilization and Reproductive Rights in America, 1950–1980*

Jennifer Lisa Koslow, *Cultivating Health: Los Angeles Women and Public Health Reform*

Jennifer Lisa Koslow, *Exhibiting Health: Public Health Displays in the Progressive Era*

Susan C. Lawrence, *Privacy and the Past: Research, Law, Archives, Ethics*

Bonnie Lefkowitz, *Community Health Centers: A Movement and the People Who Made It Happen*

Ellen Leopold, *Under the Radar: Cancer and the Cold War*

Barbara L. Ley, *From Pink to Green: Disease Prevention and the Environmental Breast Cancer Movement*

Sonja Mackenzie, *Structural Intimacies: Sexual Stories in the Black AIDS Epidemic*

Frank M. McClellan, *Healthcare and Human Dignity: Law Matters*

Michelle McClellan, *Lady Lushes: Gender, Alcohol, and Medicine in Modern America*

David Mechanic, *The Truth about Health Care: Why Reform Is Not Working in America*

Richard A. Meckel, *Classrooms and Clinics: Urban Schools and the Protection and Promotion of Child Health, 1870–1930*

Alyssa Picard, *Making the American Mouth: Dentists and Public Health in the Twentieth Century*

Heather Munro Prescott, *The Morning After: A History of Emergency Contraception in the United States*

Sarah B. Rodriguez, *The Love Surgeon: A Story of Trust, Harm, and the Limits of Medical Regulation*

Andrew R. Ruis, *Eating to Learn, Learning to Eat: School Lunches and Nutrition Policy in the United States*

James A. Schafer Jr., *The Business of Private Medical Practice: Doctors, Specialization, and Urban Change in Philadelphia, 1900–1940*

David G. Schuster, *Neurasthenic Nation: America's Search for Health, Happiness, and Comfort, 1869–1920*

Karen Seccombe and Kim A. Hoffman, *Just Don't Get Sick: Access to Health Care in the Aftermath of Welfare Reform*

Leo B. Slater, *War and Disease: Biomedical Research on Malaria in the Twentieth Century*

Piper Sledge, *Bodies Unbound: Gender-Specific Cancer and Biolegitimacy*

Dena T. Smith, *Medicine over Mind: Mental Health Practice in the Biomedical Era*

Kylie M. Smith, *Talking Therapy: Knowledge and Power in American Psychiatric Nursing*

Matthew Smith, *An Alternative History of Hyperactivity: Food Additives and the Feingold Diet*

Paige Hall Smith, Bernice L. Hausman, and Miriam Labbok, *Beyond Health, Beyond Choice: Breastfeeding Constraints and Realities*

Susan L. Smith, *Toxic Exposures: Mustard Gas and the Health Consequences of World War II in the United States*

Rosemary A. Stevens, Charles E. Rosenberg, and Lawton R. Burns, eds., *History and Health Policy in the United States: Putting the Past Back In*

Courtney E. Thompson, *An Organ of Murder: Crime, Violence, and Phrenology in Nineteenth-Century America*

Barbra Mann Wall, *American Catholic Hospitals: A Century of Changing Markets and Missions*

Frances Ward, *The Door of Last Resort: Memoirs of a Nurse Practitioner*

Jean C. Whelan, *Nursing the Nation: Building the Nurse Labor Force*

Shannon Withycombe, *Lost: Miscarriage in Nineteenth-Century America*